Placement
in Rehabilitation

Placement
in Rehabilitation
A Career Development Perspective

Edited by

David Vandergoot, Ph.D.
Director of Placement Research
Human Resources Center

and

John D. Worrall, Ph.D.

Assistant Professor of Economics
Department of Organizational and Social Sciences
New Jersey Institute of Technology

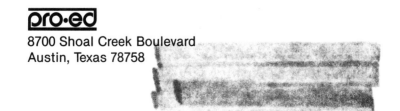

pro·ed

8700 Shoal Creek Boulevard
Austin, Texas 78758

Printed in the United States of America

Library of Congress Cataloging in Publication Data
Main entry under title:
Placement in rehabilitation.
Bibliography: p.
Includes index.
1. Handicapped — Employment — Addresses, essays,
lectures.   2. Vocational rehabilitation — Addresses,
essays, lectures.   I. Vandergoot, David.   II. Worrall,
John D.
HD7255.P56   362.8′5   79-10700
ISBN 0-936104-58-9 (previously 0-8391-1439-7)

8700 Shoal Creek Boulevard
Austin, Texas 78758

10 9 8 7 6 5   89 90 91 92 93 94

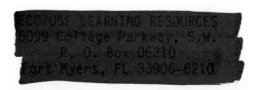

Contents

Contributors

Susanne M. Bruyère, Ph.D.
Resource and Research Specialist
Region X Rehabilitation Continuing
    Education Program
Rehabilitation Department
Seattle University
12th and East Columbia
Seattle, Washington 98122

Dennis J. Dunn, Ed.D.
Division of Rehabilitation Services
Nebraska Department of Education
301 Centennial Mall—South
Lincoln, Nebraska 68509

James Engelkes, Ph.D.
Department of Counseling,
    Personnel Services,
    and Educational Psychology
432 Erickson Hall
Michigan State University
East Lansing, Michigan 48823

Thomas W. Gannaway, Ed.D.
Director, Research and Development
Singer Education Division
80 Commerce Drive
Rochester, New York 14623

Jesse E. Gordon, Ph.D.
School of Social Work
4064 Frieze Building
The University of Michigan
Ann Arbor, Michigan 48104

Mark Granovetter, Ph.D.
Department of Sociology
State University of New York at
    Stony Brook
Stony Brook, New York 11794

David B. Hershenson, Ph.D.
Dean
Sargent College of Allied
    Health Professions
Boston University
University Road
Boston, Massachusetts 02215

Richard Jacobsen, M.A.
Research Associate
Human Resources Center
Albertson, New York 11507

**Kalisankar Mallik, M. Tech., M.S.,
Engr.**
Associate Research Professor of
    Medicine and
Director, Job Development
    Laboratory
Rehabilitation, Research, and Training
    Center
The George Washington University
420 Ross Hall
2300 Eye Street, N.W.
Washington, D.C. 20037

Carl Puleo
Executive Director
Easter Seal Goodwill Industries
    Rehabilitation Center, Inc.
20 Brookside Avenue
New Haven, Connecticut 06515

David Vandergoot, Ph.D.
Director of Placement Research
Human Resources Center
Albertson, New York 11507

William Wattenbarger, Ed.D.
Department of Counseling and Human
    Development Services
University of Georgia
Athens, Georgia 30601

John D. Worrall, Ph.D.
Director of Research
Human Resources Center
Albertson, New York 11507

Jerry J. Zadny, Ph.D.
Director, Regional Rehabilitation
    Research Institute
Portland State University
Portland, Oregon 97207

Preface

In 1977, Human Resources Center, a rehabilitation complex founded by Henry Viscardi, undertook a large-scale research project. One of the areas of concern was vocational placement in rehabilitation. As work began, it became apparent that there was little in the way of theory that could tie together all of the diverse ideas and activities that had become labeled "placement related." As study continued, it was further observed that the vocational rehabilitation process, as it is traditionally practiced, could be sharpened to better accommodate placement concerns. Existing theory and literature on labor markets was particularly helpful in suggesting a more rational way to organize the placement process in rehabilitation.

An additional concern was that vocational rehabilitation, to be successful, must open the way to long-range career development for persons with disabilities. Placement had become an end in itself and was rarely conceptualized within rehabilitation systems as a step in the long process of career development.

In response to these issues, the first chapter of this book was developed to conceptualize how vocational rehabilitation might better address the placement and career needs of people with disabilities. The practical ways of implementing these ideas were less clear. A Research Steering Committee was formed to address the problems of implementing rehabilitation services that were essential to placement and career development needs.

Individuals who are experts in various phases of the rehabilitation, placement, and career processes were invited to serve on the steering committee. Their responses to the first chapter form the remaining chapters of the book. The chapters are organized to represent a logical services sequence that suggests practical ways professionals can implement placement and career-oriented rehabilitation. Drs. Gannaway and Wattenbarger indicate the relationship between evaluation and placement activities. Dr. Hershenson describes a process that suggests the relevance of counseling for developing vocational plans. Dr. Zadny introduces the concept of developing placement plans for individuals about to begin a job search. Dr. Granovetter analyzes how information flows in the labor market and how rehabilitation professionals might capitalize on this flow to the advantage of their clients. Dr. Gordon advances a model for developing innovative approaches to job development. Dr. Engelkes describes job analysis techniques. Mr. Mallik points out in extensive detail a variety of job accommodations. Dr. Dunn deals specifically with career development variables that can lead to preparation activities while a person is still in the rehabilitation process. Mr. Puleo presents a comprehensive way of integrating employers into the rehabilitation process. Dr. Bruyère considers the difficulty that is encountered in attempting to integrate new technology, such as that presented in this book, into existing programs.

This book is intended to provide rehabilitation professionals and students with an overview of placement and career development concepts and practices. As such, it can be used to organize rehabilitation services to better meet the employment needs of people with disabilities.

Placement
in Rehabilitation

Chapter 1

New Directions for Placement Practice in Vocational Rehabilitation

David Vandergoot, Richard Jacobsen, and John D. Worrall

Recent observers of the rehabilitation scene have commented on the fragmentation of the field (Dunn 1974; Zadny and James, 1976). This state of affairs possibly arises not so much from a lack of purpose, but from confusion about how the rehabilitation of persons with disabilities can be best achieved. Often, the approach common to rehabilitation in terms of developing labor market opportunities is to rely on the goodwill of employers, emphasizing that hiring the handicapped really will not cost them very much. This approach is more like trying to find the right size Band-Aid than providing a comprehensive treatment. Practitioners in the field of rehabilitation must develop systematic procedures, based on a positive approach that helps persons with disabilities achieve success in the labor market. Optimal vocational rehabilitation will occur when the people who experience it can compete equally with others in the labor market participation. For too long rehabilitation processes have been concentrated on the final steps, which lead to placement, and have overlooked essential activities that must be taken care of long before placement is considered. Without a thorough, integrated purpose and approach, rehabilitation services focus only on temporary change. This chapter develops a comprehensive view of a rehabilitation process that places the long-range career development of the rehabilitant in mind.

The goal of placement research is to contribute to the improvement of both the quantity and quality of work available to persons with disabilities. More specifically, attempts are being made to better understand the job placement process so programs that increase employment opportunities for persons with disabilities can be designed and implemented. The primary intent of this chapter is to provide a comprehensive conceptual framework so that rehabilitation itself, as well as placement issues and processes, can be better understood.

DEFINITIONS AND DISCUSSIONS

One task of this chapter is to outline a structure for examining placement and placement-related concepts within rehabilitation. The lack of precision in many placement discussions partially stems from inconsistency in the usage of terms. In an effort to simplify the language within this book, definitions of several terms are presented. The definitions can serve both to clarify the usage of terms and to orient the reader to some of the basic concerns about placement expressed in this chapter.

Terms Relevant to Disability

The conceptual definitions presented in this chapter are borrowed from Nagi (1977). They are used with the hope that a standard set of definitions can be adopted for rehabilitation research and practice. For too long rehabilitation research has suffered because there has been no common base of reference. Nagi distinguishes four disability-related terms: pathology, impairment, functional limitation, and disability.

> *Pathology*   The state of active pathology is associated with the mobilization of defenses and coping mechanisms, and may be the result of infections, metabolic imbalances, degenerative disease processes, trauma, or other etiology.

> *Impairment*   The concept of impairment indicates a physiological, anatomical, or mental loss or other abnormality, or both . . . Examples of such impairments can be found in abnormalities and residual losses remaining after the active stage of pathology has been arrested or eliminated in non-pathological congenital deformities, and in conditions resulting from the disuse of muscle or organs for extended periods of time. Thus, although every pathology involves an impairment, not every impairment involves pathology.

> *Functional Limitations*   Functional limitations involve the level of organization at which the limitations are manifested by the organism. One could speak of limitations in function at the levels of molecules, cells, tissues, organs, regions, systems, or the organism as a whole. Although limitations at a lower level of organization may not be reflected in higher levels, the reverse is not true . . . Functional limitations at the higher levels of activities of the organism as a whole such as walking, climbing, lifting, bending, reaching, reasoning, vision, learning, correspond to what is generally referred to in the literature as a handicap.

> *Disability*   Moving beyond the level of organismic functioning to social functioning, disability has been defined as a form of inability or limitation in performing roles and tasks expected of an individual with a social environment. These tasks and roles are organized in spheres of life activities involved in self-care, education, family relations, or other interpersonal relations, recreation, economic life, and employment or vocational concerns . . . identical types of impairment and functional limitations with similar degrees of severity may result in both the reactions of the disabled and the social definition of the situation (Nagi, 1977, pp. 3–6).

As an active state, pathology will usually be of importance only to medical rehabilitation. Of central concern are the concepts of functional limitations, which result from impairment, and work disability, which results from the interaction of functional limitations with given environments. The above terms are conceptual and are not equally measurable. Pathology, impairment, and functional limitations can be directly measured against a standard; disability assessment requires consideration of the particular circumstances of an individual case. In this regard, Nagi (1977) distinguishes between operational and constitutive definitions of disability. The operational definition of disability is stated in terms of indicators and particular levels of performance. In general, pathology, impairment, and functional limitations are understood in operational terms. The constitutive definition provides the meaning of a concept in terms of other concepts; work disability is best understood and examined in this way. Adequate operational definitions of work disability are not currently available. Although vocational rehabilitation is concerned with disability as it pertains to other social roles, these role-specific disabilities are important for this chapter only insofar as they relate to work disability.

Work disability does not exist as an either/or dichotomous variable. This becomes even more apparent when considering the issue of severity. Severity is affected by aspects external to the actual impairment. These include the types of skills and abilities for productive work the individual brings to the job, the particular demands of the work site, and other factors. Thus, while the functional limitations deriving from the impairment may be permanent, the severity of the disability is seen as both impermanent and as a continuum, subject to change as circumstances are changed.

A simple example of the relative aspect of work disability can be given by looking at two persons with identical functional limitations, including limited manual strength and manual dexterity. For the manual laborer, such as a mason, the work disability deriving from this impairment may be much more severe than for a white collar administrator or salesman with the same functional limitations. Viewed in this way, the primary activities of rehabilitation can be seen as efforts to minimize the severity of work disability, which results from a given mix of circumstances. Given a permanent set of functional limitations, at least two strategies are immediately apparent. One is to alter the nature of the work environment to minimize the work barriers. Work-site modification and job restructuring are relevant here. Another approach, and this is commonly used in rehabilitation, is to alter the productivity potential the individual brings to the labor market. In this way, the interaction among individual, social, and work characteristics is rearranged.

The issue of disability and severity of functional limitation is a critical one for placement since severity is presumed to be influential in labor market exchanges. Analysis of work disability in relation to severity can suggest potential interventions. Clearly, severity contributes to different levels of employment found among persons with similar functional limitations. One of the primary tasks of research today is to develop the appropriate operational definitions of disability and severity so that they can be measured in a precise and consistent fashion. This will permit well-planned intervention. An associated problem is that most rehabilitation research has developed from the concept of impairment. The relationship between functional limitations and work disability has received limited attention.

Relevant Labor Market and Labor Force Terms

A number of labor market-related terms highly relevant to discussion of job placement and the current circumstances of persons with disabilities are defined here. The United States Bureau of the Census (1972) defines employed, unemployed, and civilian force as follows:

> *Employed*   Employed persons comprise all civilians 16 years old and over who were either: a) "at work"—those who did any work at all as paid employees or in their own business or profession, or on their own farm, or who worked 15 hours or more as unpaid workers on a family farm or in a family business; or b) were "with a job but not at work"—those who did not work during the reference week but had jobs or businesses from which they were temporarily absent due to illness, bad weather, industrial dispute, vacation, or other personal reasons.

> *Unemployed*   Persons are classified as unemployed if they were civilians 16 years old and over and: a) were neither "at work," not "with a job, but not at work" during the reference week, b) were looking for work during the past four weeks, and c) were available to accept a job. Also included as unemployed are persons who did not work at all during the reference week and were waiting to be called back to a job from which they had been laid off.

> *Civilian Labor Force*   The civilian labor force consists of persons classified as employed or unemployed in accordance with the criteria described above.

Underemployment   Even when employed, persons with disabilities may suffer from additional difficulties of underemployment in the labor market. Heneman and Yoder (1965) define underemployment as follows:

> Underemployment is the application of human resources in ways that fail to develop and use the greatest skills and potentialities that workers possess (p. 12).

Underemployment can exist in a number of ways. Persons who work part-time may be underemployed. Discriminatory practices or other factors affecting contact with the labor market, such as mobility limitations, may relegate persons to limited types of work as well as to limited income levels. Heneman and Yoder also point out an additional problem that can affect an individual's entire career development. They point to the problem of "inadequate vocational guidance and improper initial placement of younger workers who, as a result, may never have an opportunity to develop valuable aptitudes" (p. 12). Aside from reduced wages and reduced work satisfaction associated with underemployment, it is among the underemployed that unemployment increases most significantly.

Productivity   The relationship of productivity to labor market participation is reviewed in some detail shortly. In this section, suffice to say that productivity level is felt to be a critical factor determining employment in any given occupational labor market; "productivity is usually defined as 'output per man hour, quality considered'" (Heneman and Yoder, 1965, p. 11).

Career Development

Career development is a process that people use, over the course of their working lives, to receive desirable financial and nonmonetary rewards from society.

In order to develop operational definitions of career development that will facilitate research in this area, this chapter uses a concept of career development consisting of three phases: productivity enrichment, productivity realization, and career enhancement. These phases are developmental in the sense that each subsequent phase depends on the previous one; they are not, however, time-bound or limited to a certain period in a person's life. This implies that at any point in a person's work life, activities can be implemented to upgrade career development. Any attempt to contribute to career development can be classified as an activity in one of these three areas. This should help to simplify descriptions, integration, and measurement of career development activities.

Placement

The term *placement* has been used in many ways in the literature. The phrase *placement process* in rehabilitation has been applied to a series of activities by different writers, although the specific activities included are continually at issue. Discussions on where the placement process begins and ends have correspondingly identified different points in the rehabilitation process. This book presents placement as an event and not as a process. Placement is the crucial event in the rehabilitation process; it indicates that a client has accepted a job offer that yields appropriate career enhancement opportunities. Since appropriate placement is the goal of rehabilitation, all other rehabilitation activities can be related to it. In this sense, there is a rehabilitation process leading to placement, but not a distinct placement process. However, the term *placement process*, when used to focus the intent of rehabilitation services, is still a useful one.

Rehabilitation Clients

The term *client* is used frequently in this book to refer to persons with disabilities who use vocational rehabilitation services. This term has been used in the past as a subordinate description of a person involved in a relationship with a professional. This negative connotation is not intended here. Rather, the term *client* is used in the same way that Wright

(1975) uses the term *co-manager*. Rehabilitation clients are people who contribute to the development of their service delivery plan on a mutual basis with the rehabilitation professional. Rehabilitation clients are considered integral members of the rehabilitation service delivery decision-making team, and an adequate analysis of the rehabilitation process must take into account the degree to which service processes and outcomes reflect client involvement.

LABOR MARKET FACTORS

A brief overview of economic factors that affect labor market and labor force participation is presented. Rehabilitation service delivery does not exist in a vacuum. The economy that affects employment in general also affects the employment of people with disabilities.

The discussion that follows is intended to facilitate understanding of the labor market. Explanations of the concepts considered are intended to acquaint persons who are unfamiliar with the field of economics with an economic perspective. Technical jargon and complexity are kept to a minimum and examples from the field of rehabilitation are given wherever possible. Readers interested in a more sophisticated presentation are referred to Perlman (1969).

Labor Markets

The federal/state vocational rehabilitation program places most of its successful closures in the labor market, although approximately 15% of the closures are homemakers. A small percentage are placed in sheltered workshops (Rehabilitation Services Administration, 1977). A labor market consists of both buyers and sellers. Employers are buyers who demand labor, and workers are sellers who supply labor. The market is both a mechanism that allows for trades and a vehicle for allocating the human resource of labor.

There is no one labor market, although the concept is useful for discussion. There is really a series of labor markets distinguished by the extent of the market geographically or by the class or type of labor transaction that takes place in the market. Labor markets may be national or international in scope or limited to a small area. There are further discussions of types of labor markets later.

The transactions that take place in one labor market can influence what transpires in another, and this influence is strong or weak depending upon such factors as the size of the markets, the similarity of grades of labor exchanged, or the proximity of the markets. An example of this influence is the distribution of wage rates for given work. Wage rates will influence the movement of labor, and knowledge of markets will influence preparation for work and job-search activities.

The Demand for Labor

The demand for labor is a derived demand because it depends on the demand for some other good or service produced with a labor input. The demand also depends upon the productivity of labor. An employer is interested in how much more revenue an additional employee can bring to the firm. Can the employee bring revenue to the firm beyond the costs to the employer? If so, then the employee will make a contribution to the employer's profits.

Productivity is difficult to measure when the good or service produced depends upon many workers and machines. Job-searchers have different levels of productivity and the employer wants to select those who will be most productive.

An employer is concerned with what is termed the *marginal productivity* of a potential worker. Marginal productivity refers to the additional contribution in output that a new worker could provide the organization. More specifically, the marginal product of labor may be defined as the change in output resulting from a unit change in labor when all other factors in the production process are held constant.

In a profit-making organization, an employer who pays the employees a wage of greater value than what is produced will soon be out of business. This is not necessarily the case in the public sector, where there is no requirement that a firm turn a profit.

In general, however, the demand for labor will be a function of the wage rate and revenue, the productivity of labor, expected demand for the final product, technology, and social variables.

The Supply of Labor

People spend their time in either market or nonmarket activities. How this time is allocated depends on a decision made to participate or not to participate in the labor market and, given the decision to participate, on the hours of labor people are willing to supply. This decision in turn can be traced to an individual's tastes and what economists call "income and substitution effects."

Simply stated, as wages rise, leisure becomes more attractive. However, each hour spent in leisure is more expensive because time spent in nonmarket activity does not earn money. Strong empirical evidence shows that over wide ranges of the wage rate, the lure of the chance to earn is stronger than the lure of leisure. People seem to prefer to work if the wage is right. This implies that an increase in the wage rate will generally result in an increase in the hours of labor supplied.

There can be many disincentives to work for persons with disabilities. These may enable someone to maintain nonmarket activities and pursue more desirable leisure activities. Social security benefits, insurance, and other forms of nonwork income may contribute to the diminution of hours worked.

Uncertainty and Lack of Perfect Knowledge

The more knowledge buyers and sellers have about a market, the more efficiently it functions. Employers are uncertain of the future. Events occur that cannot be foreseen or predicted. In addition, employers take risks when they hire employees. They cannot precisely know an individual's productivity or potential. Hence, they may seek to minimize their risk by looking for productivity proxies in the people they hire. These might include general health, education, work and life experiences, specific or general training, or any other indices that might predict productivity. Vocational rehabilitation provides services that are productivity enriching and provide an employer with evidence that a potential employee has productive talents that can be used by the firm.

Employees also bear a risk in a labor transaction. The wage rate, which was discussed under the supply of labor, includes benefits as well as wages. A potential employee frequently does not know the conditions of employment before joining a firm. Without this knowledge, it is difficult to judge the costs associated with the effort expended in work-related activities. Generally, however, one may say that working conditions are better as wages rise.

Mistakes in the hiring process can be expensive to the employer and to the worker. The job search is costly for a worker and an employer. Turnover costs both. An employer who has trained an employee can see that investment goes down the drain should the employee quit or be discharged. Employees who take jobs that are unsuited to their skills may have wasted valuable time. Similarly, employees may take jobs that do not fully utilize their skills or do not compensate them as well as another job could. An employer may hire a worker who does not produce as well as one turned away, or no better than one who could have been hired at a lower wage. Good placements can minimize the risk for both employers and employees. Placement activity can make potential productivity a reality, minimize the costs of job search, and maximize the benefits of such a search.

Wages and Productivity

There is a direct link between an employee's productivity and the wage that an employee can command. The previous discussion pointed out that the demand for labor depends upon an employee's marginal productivity or an employer's best estimate of that marginal productivity (Levitan, Mangum, and Marshall, 1972).

In the imaginary world of perfect competition, the link between wages and productivity would also be perfect, i.e., each worker would be paid for the value of what that worker produced. Perfect competition would be characterized by many buyers and sellers, perfect knowledge (including knowledge of the future), perfect mobility of resources, devisibility of resources, and a host of other unlikely conditions and events. Labor market competition is eroded by monopolistic entities such as unions and large employers. In spite of these entities, the lack of perfect knowledge, and other factors, few people seriously challenge the link between productivity and wages.

Labor Force Decision

Before a worker can supply labor the person must decide to participate in the labor market. The wage the person expects to receive will be of critical importance in any decision about seeking employment. Having decided to participate in the labor force a job-seeker may or may not find employment at the expected wage. In such a case, expectations may be frustrated and the person may be forced to revise wage expectations downward. This process may continue until the person finds a job or withdraws from the labor market (Bowen and Finnegan, 1969).

The rehabilitation process can play a key role in this drama. It can raise the expected wage by enriching the productivity of people who use the services of the system; it can raise the actual wage that the person can receive in the labor market; it can make the job search more efficient; it can counsel a job-seeker in the actual conditions of a labor market, and give guidance on the wages and skill requirements of various jobs. It can provide job-seeking skills and information on the self-placement techniques necessary to demonstrate potential productivity to employers. The program can make nonmarket activity more expensive by making the individual with a work disability more productive.

Rehabilitation as an Investment in Human Capital

Individuals can invest in themselves. Someone could take $10,000 and place it in a savings account. That person would expect to receive a return on the $10,000 in the form of interest. Alternatively, the $10,000 could have been used to purchase a machine that manufactures skateboards. The machine would ideally be combined with labor and other inputs to produce a product that, when sold, would produce a profit. Similarly, the $10,000 could have been spent to acquire a skill, such as training as a computer programmer. Just as the "investor" in the first two examples expects a return, so too will the individual making the third investment. People who invest in themselves hope that the net increment in monetary and/or nonmonetary income discounted over a lifetime will exceed the cost of investing.

Just as individuals can invest in themselves, society can invest in people. These investments are referred to as "investments in human capital." They are designed to increase an individual's or group's productivity. Such an increase in productivity can increase an individual's or society's output. It will also raise the wage that an individual can expect to receive and, on the average, will receive (Becker, 1964).

The vocational rehabilitation program is primarily a social investment in human capital. People are not inert machines and their levels of productivity cannot be calibrated to the nearest decimal. However, logical steps can be taken to make people more productive, more attractive in the labor market, and more likely to receive higher wages.

The program is justified in part by overwhelming evidence that it does what economic theory predicts it will do. It increases the wages of the people who use its services. Most of the case services are, in fact, productivity enriching, whether or not that is the immediate intention of the client or counselor.

The rehabilitation program frequently provides what economists call general training and, occasionally, provides specific training. General training is productivity enriching and can be used in a number of different work settings. Completely specific training, while productivity enriching, increases productivity only in a specific setting and is of no value to another employer or in another setting. Distinctions between general and specific training represent a continuum and not a dichotomy. A person who has general training may leave one work setting and take the value of the training along. Employers are not as likely to provide someone with general training when the benefits of such training are likely to be absorbed by the individual trained and then easily transported away. An example of general training provided through the program would be a client who is sent to school to be an accountant. Such training is an investment in human capital and is thus of value to the person trained regardless of the accounting firm for which the trainee works.

Specific training has other implications. The rehabilitation program may have a potential selective placement in an assembly operation. If clients were trained for a specific task in the assembly operation, their productivity would be increased for a specific employer. Employers are generally willing to bear the cost of such training. Other rehabilitation services could have been chosen, medical for instance, and it would be found that they were designed, and can act, to increase productivity or to assist an individual with a work disability to realize full productive potential, i.e., employment commensurate with the person's abilities.

Placement and Realized Potential

Placement is the focus of the rehabilitation process. The rehabilitation process is designed to enrich productivity and placement is meant to ensure that the productive capacity of individuals is fully used. The placement itself is mediated by the job-search process. The act of placement and the placement process are not designed to add to a person's level of productivity. Some productivity enrichment could take place when job-seeking skills are being taught, or during the job search itself, but that is not the primary purpose of the job-search process.

The job-search process consists of activities that are designed to ensure that a client's skills are utilized as fully as possible at the best possible wage, where wage includes benefits and job conditions, given the costs of job search and the state of the labor market.

The best possible placement may not be one that fully utilizes an individual. For example, an individual could be underemployed because the local economy does not have a job opening requiring all the skills that the individual has attained. The goal then is to find the best placement within constraints of the job-search process and labor market conditions.

Primary and Secondary Labor Markets

Although some labor market analysts adhere rigorously to the belief that there are actually well-defined primary and secondary labor markets, the labor market is too complex to be divided so grossly. An understanding of the concept of dual labor markets is useful, however, in understanding the role placement can play in career development.

Primary labor markets are generally characterized by occupations that provide relatively high wages, excellent working conditions, on-the-job training, productivity-enriching activities, and a job ladder. Secondary labor markets represent occupations that are not likely to provide on-the-job training or an opportunity for advancement. Productivity enrichment in this market could actually be negative, because job holders acquire work habits and attitudes that lead to lower productivity (see Freiman, 1976).

Ideally, placement, as defined above, should result in the optimum use of a person's skills over a period of time. When possible, people should be placed in positions with a possibility for growth and continuing productivity enrichment. Those who use rehabilitation placement services and those who provide them must realize that the type of position the client is placed in will play a role in subsequent career development. The client should not necessarily be placed in the first available position. Issues involved in making placement decisions will be discussed more fully within the context of developing job openings and within the context of evaluating the long-range potential of a given job offer.

THE REHABILITATION PROCESS: A CONCEPTUAL OVERVIEW

Job Placement Overview

In discussing the job placement process, those factors that enable people to successfully prepare for, find, and keep jobs that they want are a main concern. In rehabilitation, three processes have been noted: 1) preparation for a job, 2) finding a job, and 3) keeping a job. Agencies involved with placement as it is outlined here may in practice and in intent address themselves to any combination of these three. Some agencies may concentrate exclusively on preparation for employment or even on a particular aspect of preparation (e.g., physical therapy). Another program may be organized primarily around assistance in finding a job. The federal/state vocational rehabilitation system is a comprehensive program in that all three processes are within its service range. The fact that all of these exist together and are, in general, served by the same staff leads to a blurring of the functions involved and a confusion in roles and service needs. This is particularly evident in the ongoing debates in the field regarding counselors' roles in placement.

Whether a comprehensive program exists from the agency's perspective, the ideal placement program will substantially increase the individual's productivity potential through vocational skill development. The gain derived from skill development will enable individuals to expand the range of concrete work choices available to them in the labor market. Thus placement involves both the enrichment of the individual's productivity potential and the nature of a person's contact with the labor market during the job search. A tremendous number of factors impinge on the capacity of any placement-directed service program to fulfill both of these requirements. The focus of this chapter is the identification of these requirements within a coherent, conceptual framework.

Job placement has long been a focal point of discussion in rehabilitation and has been the topic of many writings, as well as an overriding concern of many model programs. Unfortunately, many of these efforts are repetitive or contradictory and the value of any given model, although it may be great, remains unclear. Recently, two major reviews of the literature on job placement in rehabilitation have been conducted

(Dunn, 1974; Zadny and James, 1976). Each has included overall comments on placement literature. Dunn, in his preface, remarks:

> Once I started reviewing the literature, it quickly became obvious that there is a vast amount of literature available on placement and to review it all would be a tedious and perhaps thankless chore. It was also obvious that much of it was repetitious. It also seemed fragmented and unattached to anything (p. i).

In a similar vein, Zadny and James (1976) comment in their introduction:

> The abundance of writings on placement in vocational rehabilitation attests to an accumulated wisdom and sophistication which is not borne out by careful inspection of the materials and is clearly contradicted in practice. ... Beyond the facade of sheer volume there is little sense of real progression marked by notions challenged and proven with newer developments built on old ... the literature has proliferated unrestrained by burdens of proof and requirements of synthesis. Therefore, placement remains genuinely an art; each practitioner selecting from the many methods known on the basis of preference and taste (pp. 1–2).

It need not be inferred from these comments that the literature in placement is without value. The form that the literature has taken, however, makes it difficult to systematically study what is known, what remains unknown, or even the questions being asked. Consequently, the literature offers only limited guidance to people involved in placement or to people attempting to organize placement programs.

The fragmentation in the literature appears to stem from many sources. Part of the problem in developing consistency in placement discussions is that placement relates to virtually all phases of rehabilitation, leading to a tremendous diversity of perspectives on the subject.

In state vocational rehabilitation programs, for example, phases in the rehabilitation process include intake, evaluation, service planning, and service provisions—including physical restoration services, counseling and guidance, skill training, placement, and post-employment services. When investigated more closely each of these phases breaks down into a multitude of concerns, needs, and interactions that can affect placement outcomes.

Thus, a tremendous splintering occurs when each of these sub-areas is investigated. A number of other factors further complicate discussion. One is the issue of whether or not a given agency is structured to encourage placement as an outcome. This issue poses methodological as well as organizational questions.

Accompanying this diversity in placement issues and perspectives has been continuing uncertainty over the appropriate roles and functions of rehabilitation professionals. Much of this concern has focused on the role of the counselor. Whitten (1975), in a historical overview of the rehabilitation counselor's role since the 1940s, notes an expansion of counseling duties and an associated reduction in the coordinator-type functions often associated with job placement. Consistent with this trend, Salomone (1971) has advocated the "client-centered" approach to placement, in which the counselor is primarily responsible for helping clients to find jobs on their own. Distancing counselors from placement activities is supported by advocates of placement specialists (Lillehaugen, 1964; Hutchinson and Cogan, 1974) within the rehabilitation system, who would relieve the counselor of many placement functions.

Others (Hart and Karbott, 1964; Echols, 1972; Flannagan, 1974) argue that the actual placement process should not be separated from the earlier portions of the rehabilitation process, which are geared to develop readiness to compete in the labor market. Usdane (1974, 1976), in supporting the concept of a professional placement worker, feels that many counselors are insufficiently trained to meet the demands of professional placement work and calls for a graduate school curriculum to fulfill this need.

The debate over placement's role reflects, on the one hand, a tendency for counselors to be the people most interested in counseling due to their training experiences. On the other hand, agencies are predominately concerned with job placement as a service outcome rather than with counseling as a process. Zadny and James (1976) indicate that their review of the literature led them to conclude that the "counselor is held accountable for an outcome without being advised on how to secure quality results" (p. 4). This is a dilemma that could contribute to feelings of frustration and therefore detract from the professionalism of rehabilitation counselors. If this is so, the lack of a comprehensive theoretical framework integrating placement within the rehabilitation process could contribute to serious confusion. Ehrle (1969) has suggested that counselor turnover could result from agency operations and from professional issues that reflect this type of conflict. The consequent loss of valuable professional expertise and initiative represents a corresponding loss of rehabilitation services within the rehabilitation setting. This argument is continued by Sussman and Haug (1970), who present research suggesting that deprofessionalization is a problem in rehabilitation counseling.

The issues outlined here have implications for both the rehabilitation counseling profession and for the type of comprehensive service approach possible within the rehabilitation system. The functions of professionals within the vocational rehabilitation system and the organization of programs should logically derive from a theoretical understanding of a placement-oriented rehabilitation program. Given a set of agreed-upon needs and processes in an effective, comprehensive placement program, the delineation of professional roles and services becomes more immediately an organizational, and not a theoretical, concern. If specific needs for placement are identified, rehabilitation activities and services can be geared to meet them. The goal of this chapter is to begin the development of a reconceptualization of the rehabilitation process that would permit a systematic approach to overcoming work disabilities. Examining the rehabilitation process in light of the labor market principles previously reviewed in this chapter can facilitate a better understanding of service delivery needs and program organization.

A Reconceptualization of the Rehabilitation Process

In the review of labor market principles, the productivity level of workers stands out as a significant matter in rehabilitation. This review led to a discussion of the relationship of productivity levels to hiring. The importance of adequate planning for productivity, based on a comprehensive knowledge of skill requirements, was indicated.

With the achievement of given productivity, placement is sought at the highest possible level during the job search. Looking at the placement situation, two distinct processes can be identified that enable a person to obtain satisfactory employment: 1) the enrichment of levels of productivity potential so that the person can compete in the primary labor market and 2) the productivity realization process, including the job-search process and actual placement. The job-search process is directed toward ensuring that the person's productivity potential is fully realized in the job by bringing the highest return possible in monetary and nonmonetary income for the individual's investment in productivity enrichment.

Efforts to upgrade the participation level of persons with disabilities in the labor market can be seen with respect to these two processes—productivity enrichment and productivity realization—through the job search and subsequent placement.

Within rehabilitation programs the comprehensive service approach devotes considerable attention to both of these processes. Many activities currently seen in rehabilitation can be understood from this perspective, and various service needs or gaps can be recognized as well. Rehabilitation services that are productivity enriching include, but are not limited to, skill training to increase productivity and efforts to reduce obstacles to productivity (such as counseling, assistance in development of mobility, and assistance in obtaining prosthetic or orthotic devices). Productivity enrichment activities, proceeding from evaluations of previously developed productivity levels, are designed to further enhance the labor market positions of clients.

Once a person has participated in a variety of productivity-enriching activities, the productivity realization phase takes over; the job search and active placement occur. The job-search activities of a client, a counselor, or any other person or agency, seek to maximize a person's employment level at the least possible cost.

While productivity enrichment, job search, and placement have been discussed generally in the context of an initial placement through rehabilitation services, these factors continue to operate throughout a person's participation in the labor market and throughout career development in general. A person's career development will continue to reflect the relationship between productivity levels and job opportunities. Related issues that are also important in the job search are the potential costs and benefits of job mobility. The career development process, therefore, includes productivity enrichment, productivity realization, and career enhancement. Figure 1 highlights these processes and notes a few of the many factors affecting the general environment for vocational rehabilitation. Rehabilitation programs contribute to each of these three processes during a limited period of time in a person's overall career development, although they focus primarily on the first two. Service delivery activities can be understood in terms of their impact on these processes, and, in the long run, on the career development of each client.

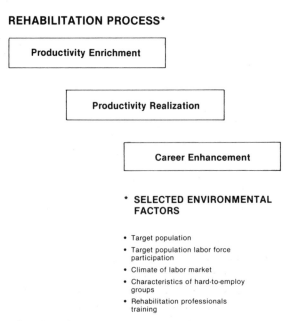

REHABILITATION PROCESS*

> **Productivity Enrichment**

> **Productivity Realization**

> **Career Enhancement**

* SELECTED ENVIRONMENTAL FACTORS

- Target population
- Target population labor force participation
- Climate of labor market
- Characteristics of hard-to-employ groups
- Rehabilitation professionals training

Figure 1.   Overview of the rehabilitation process and selected factors affecting it.

Therefore, all rehabilitation services become meaningful to the client since it can be shown how services contribute to career development.

Rehabilitation service agencies currently work within these frameworks of productivity enrichment and productivity realization, although they are not generally thought of as doing so. The implied relationship of these activities to career development needs to be stated more directly. Naturally, many subprocesses go on within these phases (productivity enrichment, productivity realization, and career enhancement), and they are the basis of many of the issues currently discussed in the rehabilitation and placement literature. Clarification of the relationship of these various activities to the overall rehabilitation process will provide meaning and direction to the service activities of rehabilitation counselors and will contribute to the clarity of their professional roles and status. Applying the economically derived perspective of rehabilitation services also permits an identification of the roles employers, rehabilitation clients, and general community resources can play in the process.

Finally, this concept of the rehabilitation process clarifies the goal of service programs and indicates what they can be held accountable for. Rehabilitation services exist so that people with disabilities can obtain jobs that maximize the return on their own and society's investment in the enrichment of their productivity potential. As the quality of rehabilitation services continues to improve, people with disabilities should enter primary labor markets to a much greater extent.

Thus, the remainder of this section is divided into three major segments:

A. Discussion of the productivity enrichment processes, including:
   1. developing information
   2. developing strategy for productivity enrichment
   3. strategy implementation for productivity enrichment
B. Discussion of the productivity realization (or job search and placement) activities, including:
   1. developing a job-search strategy
      a. identifying factors affecting job search activity
      b. identifying the appropriate sources of labor market information for search activities
      c. accessing the labor market, including both locating and developing job openings
   2. obtaining the placement
C. Discussion of career enhancement, including follow-up and job maintenance activities, as well as general factors in career enhancement

Although these processes as outlined here appear to be discrete activities, they are all interrelated. One does not begin where another ends. The outline does, however, convey a general sequence of what might be a major activity at any point in the rehabilitation process. For example, skills assessment should occur first in the process, but strategy development and implementation activities might also occur at the same time to some extent. This section also highlights how employers can participate in and contribute to the rehabilitation process. Not enough attention has been paid to the diverse functions employers can perform.

It must be emphasized that throughout the rehabilitation process, from information-seeking to follow-up, the counselor is responsible for establishing and maintaining a psychological climate that permits the development of a working counseling relationship. Counseling skills facilitate the necessary give-and-take that encourages maximum client participation in rehabilitation. This type of counseling relationship will increase the impact rehabilitation services have on the career development of clients.

Productivity Enrichment

Developing Information   The rehabilitation process attempts to provide disabled persons with the productivity levels necessary to enter the labor market. Therefore, the process begins with productivity enrichment activities. Figure 2 provides an overview of the productivity enrichment phase and highlights a few processes that affect enrichment activities. The first activity leading to this is developing information.

Information development begins with an appraisal of the quality of a client's general and specific skills to determine what needs, if any, still exist in these areas. This process is an enlargement of the traditional work readiness assessment commonly used. Since productivity enrichment is a process begun during a person's early years, educational experience is a crucial contributor. The role that productivity enrichment plays in subsequent career development highlights the need for a quality education that provides youngsters who have disabilities with a thorough career orientation. A good part of a person's early life, including educational and vocational training and experience, can be described as a process providing general skills that can be applied to the basic requirements of a wide spectrum of potential occupations. Usually attention is not paid to specific occupational training until a person begins to think about obtaining a job. This initial needs assessment must take into account information that involves a wide variety of sources. The client must participate with the counselor in developing a suitable knowledge base from which decisions can be made and strategies determined. The counselor must direct this information-seeking activity and maintain the

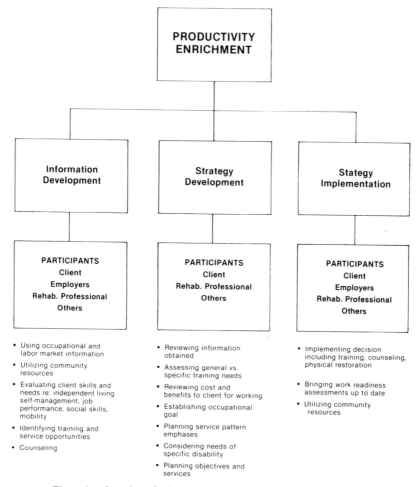

Figure 2.   Overview of selected processes in productivity enrichment.

role of expert. The client must participate in giving and developing the information, which will be needed to sufficiently plan for rehabilitation services. The following psychosocial areas need to be assessed:

1. Education skills
2. Community living skills
3. Independent living skills
4. Self-management skills, including self-placement skills
5. Career development knowledge

This assessment process can employ data obtained in numerous ways. Educational and medical reports can be examined. A psychological assessment can be used to integrate the personal and emotional needs of the client with developing a rehabilitation plan. Community resources can be used by the client and counselor alike to gather information regarding such things as transportation, social service, and employment support. Employers can play a particularly important role in providing labor market information to the counselor and world-of-work exposure to the client.

World-of-work information must encompass national and local employment. The client must become as familiar as possible with occupations and types of jobs within occupations. Entry-level skills and skills for advancement need to be evaluated in light of the costs to obtain them and the benefits to be derived from having them. Educational and training opportunities need to be considered and, most important of all, the demand for various occupations must be determined. Although it is important not to limit one client to a certain geographical area, client mobility needs and social ties may dictate that a certain region is preferable. World-of-work information must be tailored to this chosen region. The local labor market and economy must be understood. Jobs that are lasting and provide career enhancement opportunities need to be identified.

Strategy Development   The skills assessment process forms the basis for developing strategies, which begins the second stage of productivity enrichment. Informed decisions are used to determine the direction of productivity enrichment activities, which will further prepare the client to compete in a given labor market. Developing strategies begins with setting goals that indicate which occupation and labor market meets the needs and skill potential of the client. This implies that the counselor and client have thoroughly reviewed and integrated the relevant information. Dunn (1974) has stated that a "shortcoming within the current vocational rehabilitation program is the lack of emphasis upon client careers. Traditionally, not much attention has been paid to the long run" (p. 25). This can be remedied by a careful consideration of the client's personal characteristics, particularly skill potential and needs, and how the world of work can permit skills to be used and needs fulfilled in a way that will result in satisfying careers. Vocational information cannot be overemphasized. Rehabilitation practitioners have access to various forms of work evaluation; these can be particularly helpful means of providing clients with the opportunity to gain vocational information and to integrate it as they experience the process. Information derived from work evaluation can be particularly meaningful and real to clients.

The long-range employment goal can be subdivided into components that express the client's desired personal, social, and leisure needs; these can be used to reinforce the client's efforts to achieve career enhancement. Typical decision-making strategies suggest that, following the choice of a long-range goal, alternatives should be generated, possibly by brainstorming techniques (D'Zurrilla and Goldfried, 1971), which have the potential for contributing to goal accomplishment. Appropriate objectives can then be chosen and steps taken to reach the objectives. The counselor and client can each have responsibility for accomplishing steps.

To facilitate decision-making that will lead to an appropriate enrichment of the client's productivity level, factors other than skills must also be considered. Personal characteristics, such as the ability to get along with co-workers and supervisors, and the need for supportive medical services and assistive devices are important. Client self-management, such as maintaining time schedules, finances, and proper nutrition, is also important. Environmental characteristics, such as the presence or absence of technological and architectural modifications, transportation, and other community resources and social supports must be considered. These must be viewed as factors that affect the productivity potential of the client. While skills are essential to productivity, complications that could act as limits to productivity need to be identified.

Long-range goals for the rehabilitation process must indicate the type of placement available to the client that will permit the potential for enhancement of the client's career. Once a suitable long-range goal is decided upon, specific strategies for reaching the goal can be developed. Further decisions must be made regarding the intermediate objectives and learning activities the client must pursue. Again, the counselor must act as a guide and resource person for the client as the strategy evolves. In order to form these intermediate objectives, the information pool must again be used. New information may be needed if there are not sufficient data for making decisions. Intermediate objectives must be based on the relevance they have for meeting the client's ultimate placement goal, and strategies dictated by intermediate objectives must lead to that goal. The information describing client characteristics and relevant world-of-work factors can serve as a basis for deciding what productivity levels the client has previously achieved and to see what still has to be achieved. The activities pursued to reach intermediate objectives can all enrich client productivity. These include not only vocational training and education, but also traditional rehabilitation services, such as work and personal adjustment training, counseling, medical and physical restoration services, and any other activity that can potentially better prepare a client for suitable placement. There is no limit to the types of activity that contribute to productivity enrichment. Creativity is at a premium during strategy development.

Any of these strategies can be viewed as investments in human capital (Becker, 1964). In other words, productivity enrichment can be described as an investment in human resources, yielding both monetary income and nonmonetary income. Investment can include any of these services as long as they can potentially "improve skills, knowledge, or health, and, thereby, raise money or psychic income" (Becker, 1964, p. 1).

Strategy Implementation   Once strategies have been created to determine the steps and activities needed to meet objectives and the ultimate placement goal, the third productivity enrichment stage, strategy implementation, can begin. At this point the client attempts to enrich and increase productivity. The strategy plan must be properly sequenced and intermediate outcomes must be described in advance so that responsibilities and expectations are clear to both client and counselor. This also affords a careful assessment of progress and sufficient opportunity for revision if the plan is deficient. To help assess progress, rehabilitation counselors can use work readiness concepts to see whether or not the client exhibits suitable general skills to enter the chosen labor market. If not, further general preparation in the form of work adjustment training may be needed. If specific skill training is a part of the client's productivity enrichment plan, then the skills developed through training by the client must be evaluated in terms of what the specific job requires. On-the-job training can be a valuable assessment tool and is another important area in which employers can play a crucial role by making opportunities available to clients. In this way employers can participate in strategy accomplishment. This involvement on the part of the employers can also be used to introduce them to technological and architectural modifications that permit the hiring of persons with disabilities. By making these modifications, employers make a major contribution to the career development process.

The counselor and client must carefully consider the blend of general and specific training that a client receives during productivity enrichment. General training is important, but specific training for a particular job might improve the client's relative standing in the labor market and increase the wage the client could expect in that particular labor market.

"Rational firms pay generally trained employees the same wage and specifically trained employees a higher wage than they could get elsewhere" (Becker, 1964, p. 24); hence, on-the-job training, if available, seems desirable. Workshop and rehabilitation center training may be valuable only insofar as it provides general training. Specific training in these settings may not be as efficient as the specific training provided by an actual firm. The quality of rehabilitation service can be monitored by eventually assessing the financial and nonmonetary incomes a person receives due to productivity enrichment. This again indicates the importance of integrating labor market knowledge into the rehabilitation plan. Knowing what occupations are or will be in demand will enable the plan to incorporate the specific training that will increase the return of investment in productivity enrichment. Specific training highlights the relevance of accurate vocational guidance to eventual ability to compete in a labor market characterized by technological advance and skill upgrading. It must also be remembered that many strategies, besides the obvious vocational training experience described here, contribute to the client's productivity enrichment. Counseling, physical restoration, medical and maintenance services, family services, remedial education, and any other services that enrich clients as human resources to themselves and to society are valid productivity enrichment activities. When it is determined that the strategy for productivity enrichment has been completed to the fullest extent possible through rehabilitation services, the counselor and client can move on to productivity realization and develop a job-search strategy.

Productivity Realization

Introduction   Throughout the productivity enrichment phase of the rehabilitation process, investments are made in the individual's capability to compete in the labor market. Investments are made by the individual with the disability, by the counselor(s) involved in the process, by the agency, and by many others, such as family, friends, or local community resources. The goal of the productivity realization phase of the rehabilitation process is to ensure that the return from these investments to the individual and society is maximized. Thus maximization begins when the job is obtained and, eventually, in the career enhancement made possible by that job.

The productivity realization phase includes activities that lead to an appropriate placement. Many concerns become apparent here. What motivates the job-search effort? What effect on the client do financial disincentives have? What strategy should the client employ? What is the role of the counselor? What are the employer's attitudes toward persons with disabilities? What are employers' recruitment and screening practices? How important are job-seeking skills? Clearly, much of the placement literature, as it is traditionally classified, can be examined in terms of this realization process. Additional concepts from other fields can be drawn upon to enhance current understandings.

The conceptual model used to distinguish productivity enrichment from productivity realization provides a means of identifying relationships among concepts and points of contribution or dissent within the literature and in practice. It is nonetheless recognized that the rehabilitation process is ongoing; the distinction made here between productivity enrichment and productivity realization is not always clear in practice.

For instance, in the case of an on-the-job training program, both productivity enrichment and productivity realization may be achieved. This, of course, is part of the appeal of such a program.

Productivity realization is a process that culminates when a job-seeker accepts a job. The process itself consists of three related activities. These activities are intended to develop a job-search strategy and include:

1. Identifying factors that will affect an individual's job-search motivation
2. Identifying the appropriate sources of labor market information for search activities
3. Making the labor market accessible, including locating and developing job openings

Figure 3 provides a schematic representation of these processes in productivity realization. A proper integration of the information obtained through these activities should permit an individual to accept a

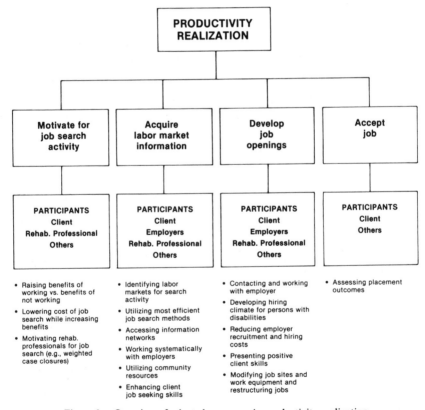

Figure 3.   Overview of selected processes in productivity realization.

job offer that begins the lifelong process of maximizing productivity enrichment investments. Accepting a job initiates the placement event. The productivity realization process presented here is a general framework describing factors and activities that need to be considered when searching for employment. How they are used with individuals in the counseling process depends on the unique circumstances of the persons involved.

Identification of Factors Affecting Job-Search Activity   Factors that affect job-search activity begin during the stage of productivity enrichment. The period of productivity enrichment involves various rehabilitation services, including skill training, that function to increase a person's standing in a labor market. Ideally, an individual becomes more desirable as an employee through productivity enrichment. This will better enable a person to successfully find a satisfactory job in the primary labor market at higher pay. It also provides a stronger chance for career enhancement independent of further rehabilitation services. The labor market advantages derived from the period of productivity enrichment can raise the benefits of employment and correspondingly increase the cost of nonparticipation in the labor force.

The costs and benefits of labor force participation are also important to job-search activity. It is useful, as suggested by job-search theory, to examine the costs and benefits to a person participating in the labor force. Likewise, it will be instructive to examine the relative costs of the job search for the individual.

Kasper (1967) notes that the income (monetary or nonmonetary) of working must be sufficient to compensate for the lost benefits of not working. Some potential benefits of not working include the flexible leisure time and the relative freedom of not working. Within rehabilitation, the concept of "secondary gains" of disability has also been discussed in relation to the motivation to search for and take a job. Secondary gains refer to the relative advantages of the sick or disabled role. Nagi and Hadley (1972) note such benefits as "the ability to control the actions of others, the receipt of emotional support, and the satisfaction of dependency inclinations" (p. 223).

Another issue, and the issue to which Nagi and Hadley apply their research, is that of financial disincentives and work motivation among persons with disabilities. Nagi and Hadley (1972) examined relationships among disability and income levels, focusing on income change following the onset of disability. In some cases, the cost of disability is offset by supplementary support incomes. In other cases, a substantial income loss was sustained. Data reported support the idea that motivation to work is not as affected by absolute income levels as it is by the relative cost of disability to the individual. If income levels are substantially reduced following the onset of disability, motivation to work appears to be greater, except among those with severe limitations. If overall income levels remain relatively stable due to various forms of compensation or new earnings resulting from another family member entering the labor market, work motivation is not great. This research on income change highlights the importance of attending to the relative costs and benefits of working and of disability. Anticipated costs and benefits could affect both job-search behavior and the asking wage a person uses to guide the search.

If productivity enrichment succeeds in increasing the wage a person can expect, that person will also be more likely to enter the labor market, since relative benefits of working increase. The relative benefits of working also increase as the individual is able to make the optimal choice in the labor market. There is an additional problem that compounds the cost/benefit estimates of labor force participation: imperfect and incomplete information. The client seeking a job wants to maximize the return on the investment in productivity enrichment, and this maximization is usually accomplished in the labor market. Labor markets operate to distribute human resources and consist essentially of buyers and sellers of labor. Employers seeking workers and, in this case, clients looking for work hope to strike the best possible bargain. The client wants to find the best job possible at the best wage possible. Unfortunately, the job-seeking client cannot have a complete knowledge of the available job markets, and is not assured of making the best job choice. In order to choose well, the job-seeker wants to have the proper information about job openings and wage rates. Since this is impossible, the job-seeker must estimate what might be expected in the labor market. Costs for obtaining information must not become prohibitive, and, for this reason alone, estimates are essential. McCall (1970) suggests that a job-seeker will have estimates of the wage distribution for particular skills, and will continue to search until an offer consistent with these expectations is made. It is likely that a person's estimate may be adjusted when information is obtained about the circumstances of the labor market or as job offers at given wage rates develop or fail to develop.

Information becomes critical to the job-seeker, however, when making estimates of justified asking prices. McCall (1970) notes that a person may overestimate or underestimate the wage that can be commanded. If the client underestimates both job and wage and settles for a job that is below legitimate productivity levels, full return on the first portions of the rehabilitation process is not obtained. If the job-seeking client overestimates job and wage possibilities, the cost and time invested in the job search might be wasted. In some cases, the individual might drop out of the labor market feeling discriminated against or finding the job search too costly; then the full investment in productivity enrichment may be lost, both for the client and the rehabilitation agency. The person who has realistic, competent knowledge of the labor market will be less likely to underestimate or overestimate opportunities. Job offers are a basic source of wage rate information. The more job offers a person is able to locate and develop, the greater the opportunity to make the optimal choice.

To summarize, several factors have been identified that affect a person's job-search activity. These include the person's investment in productivity enrichment, the costs and benefits of labor force participation for that person, the relative costs of the job search, and imperfect and incomplete knowledge about the labor market. The counselor and client must carefully consider the impact these factors may have, seek to identify the appropriate labor markets, and locate available information.

Identification of Appropriate Sources of Labor Market Information

At this stage of the process, information for the job search is crucial. Information on the labor market might be gained in a variety of ways. Job-search methods commonly cited include reviewing newspaper ads and trade journals, visiting state and private employment agencies, making direct application to businesses, asking friends and relatives, and reviewing written materials. However, methods of job search vary in at least two major respects: 1) the efficiency of the methods in obtaining desired labor market information and job offers and 2) the costs of the search for the information. Research (Jaffe, Day, and Adams, 1964; Sheppard and Belitsky, 1966; Jones and Azrin, 1973) indicates that some sources of job leads have been more effective in the past than others. It may well be that job-seekers frequently invest poorly in their job search through inaccurate estimates of the most effective job-search methods. Friends and relatives and direct application to a company are most effective of all.

Even given an accurate assessment of efficient job-search methods, what investments of time and other resources must be made to obtain labor market information? Costs include transportation costs, the purchase of materials, telephone expenses, foregone leisure time, and psychological costs. The cost of obtaining information may be greater than the individual is willing to invest.

With respect to persons with impairments, this becomes a particularly challenging concern; although the principle of attempting to maximize the return from job-search investments remains, the impairment may alter the balance of cost and benefit. For instance, one way to search for jobs and job information, particularly job offers, is to get on the phone and call people. For the deaf person, it may be that the cost of making an identical number of contacts is much greater than it is for someone who is not deaf. General attitudes toward persons with disabilities might also affect the effectiveness and cost of search methods.

The cost of the job search will also be related to the cost of taking a job. These combined costs may induce a person to drop out of the labor market without obtaining a job. McCall (1970) comments:

> The search policy when people with unattractive employment opportunities are confronted with relatively high information costs may be to choose the null occupation, i.e. to choose not to search for alternative employment (p. 114).

This phenomenon further demonstrates the importance for the jobseeker of obtaining maximum knowledge about the immediate labor market at the lowest cost possible. Specifically, the job-seeker needs to know where offers are available and what wages are associated with them. Therefore, rehabilitation processes geared toward maximizing returns from productivity enrichment investments will seek to both maximize labor market information (including information leading to job offers) and lower the cost of that information during the productivity realization phase.

The job search also involves costs for the counselor. Within the current state/federal vocational rehabilitation system, the 26 closure does not take the quality of the placement into consideration. Currently, the benefits of a placement to the counselor are largely unaffected either by the difficulty or the quality of the placement; this provides limited motivation for the counselor to engage in sustained job-search activities on behalf of clients. Discussions and research in the area of weighted case closures are attempts to address the problem. The potential value of increasing counselor benefits with relation to job placement efforts remains to be seen.

Specifically, the type of information needed to maximize returns from the job search concerns the labor market. The decision process must compare one job offer with others that might be expected, taking into account how available offers are and where they are located. An understanding of labor markets is essential.

Heneman and Yoder (1965) point out three types of labor markets useful for analysis: 1) geographical, 2) occupational (labor market for a given occupation, e.g., accountants, typists, instructional writers), and 3) industrial (such as steel, agricultural). A person needs to decide which labor markets are to be considered possibilities for employment. With respect to geographical markets, how far is a person willing or able to travel? Mobility difficulties for persons with disabilities can be relevant here, as well as level of independent living skills. A person can expand available labor markets by a willingness or ability to be mobile.

With respect to occupational labor markets, the person needs to decide on a desirable, specific job. This idea could be expanded to include related jobs. The person needs to be aware of various options within job titles and classifications that might be satisfactory. Unawareness of related occupations and occupational titles can restrict a person's job search, leaving potentially fertile labor markets unexplored. In this sense, a person wants to intensify the job search by investigating all possible areas.

Gaining Access to the Labor Market—Locating and Developing Job Openings Once the needed areas of information have been identified, a strategy can be developed to obtain the information. Labor market information, which identifies potential work areas, can form the basis in developing a strategy for collecting specific information about what jobs are available and what job offers might develop. Ideally, much of this information will also have formed the basis in service planning for productivity enrichment. Then the job search becomes a further application of this information and not an unrelated rehabilitation activity. Occupational information clearly can continuously contribute to the rehabilitation process.

The organization of a community can affect informal communication or information networks. Krippendorf (1971) argues that communication as a process leads to the development of social structure and to patterned interactions, or networks. Persons or organizations involved in various types of exchange activities encourage communication. Various activities lead to personal or organizational interactions relevant to the business at hand. A network through which information can pass easily is then developed. Two businessmen in a given industry or occupation will be more likely to exchange business-related information than information about pottery making. However, if they are meeting at a convention of pottery enthusiasts, different communication patterns and networks will be used, leading to a different type of information exchange.

Today's society is highly integrated and information can pass quickly through these information networks if properly recognized and assessed. Previous work (Coleman, Katz, and Menzel, 1957; Katz, 1957; Lee, 1969; Granovetter, 1974) demonstrates the role of information networks in promoting social action. In his study of job-finding, Granovetter (1974) introduces his orientation, based on information network assumptions:

> I will be pursuing the findings of earlier studies which indicated that information which leads to action is more likely to move through chains of personal contact than through mass media or more impersonal routes (p. 4).

What is critical is an understanding of the structural factors that lead to the association of persons and to the consequent development of information networks. With this understanding, desired information can be more easily obtained.

Labor markets, as noted earlier, are organized in at least three significant ways: by geography, by occupation, and by industry. Knowing this should help in planning initial approaches to relevant information networks for gaining labor market information. This in turn can both expand contacts in information networks and lead to job offers. The shapes, types, and magnitude of labor markets will help indicate strategies in job search, as will the level of job sought. Granovetter (1974) also suggests that to a large degree the critical information is not reserved only for close friends, as one might suspect, but is generally available to any interested person.

Important here also is the notion that the manner in which information is solicited is critical to the type of information received. This communication will structure the type of response made and the information received. The most informed approach to a question will tend to receive the most informed response. This notion is important because the job-seeker may inadvertently miss some key information by not being able to accurately pose a question. Implications for the job-search activities of the rehabilitation professional, for job search counseling, and for the activities of the client involved in job search are clear. Strategies point toward development of as much information as is possible and reasonable, given costs and needs. This information will assist in making the optimal decision in the job search and help ensure the best possible placement. Strategies for developing this information need to be further researched.

Relevant also to strategies for developing and locating job offers is an understanding of employer search patterns. The employer will also be interested in locating the best employee at the least search cost and at the lowest realistic wage. In addition, the employer will be uncertain of the range of potential workers available and the wage they will be willing to accept.

In the primary labor market, the employer tends to have a relatively fixed wage rate range, and this range serves as a consistent signal to job-seekers who estimate their market worth to be in that range (Lippman and McCall, 1976). Having solicited job-seeking response within this range, the employer will be concerned with the productivity of the applicants and the contributions to the organization's production that the potential worker, if hired, can make. The employer must decide how much can be gained from hiring one person rather than another. The employer will also need to decide if the costs of continued searching and foregone production will make waiting for still other job applicants too expensive. Thus, the employer is involved in making estimates of a potential worker's productivity. Lippman and McCall (1976) point out the difficulties job-searchers have in transmitting information about their productivity level to searching employers.

Employers will be attentive to factors that they believe are associated with productivity levels. Spence (1973) distinguishes between two classifications of traits believed to be associated with productivity: indices and signals. Indices are unalterable attributes, such as race or sex. In rehabilitation-related placement, an index would be the impairment of the individual. Signals are observable characteristics, such as education or training, that can change and are subject to manipulation by the individual.

When measuring a job applicant's expected productivity level, assessments can be influenced by both indices and signals. Certain signals will be associated in the employer's mind with higher or lower productivity levels. The job-seeker will attempt to highlight those market signals the employer might feel are negatively associated with productivity. Many job-seeking skills programs, which have demonstrated success in aiding job-finding (McClure, 1972; Keith, 1976), focus on the job-seeker's ability in the job interview to effectively present productivity-related signals (e.g., work histories, work skills, education, training). Literature on selective placement activities by the counselor (McDonald, 1974) also focuses on counselor advocacy of client skills. Advocacy in this area can best be accomplished through an understanding of those signals that employers view as productivity related. This same understanding can guide service planning in productivity enrichment and should be made specific to employers' job needs and concerns.

The employer will also tend to assess productivity on the basis of indices, even though these assessments are not necessarily accurate. Race and sex discrimination arguments focus on this question. Similarly, employer attitudes and lack of knowledge regarding the work capabilities of persons with disabilities can constitute a significant barrier to employment. In this context it is important for rehabilitation professionals to develop a climate for hiring. Job development activities are potentially significant in this regard. An aim of the productivity realization phase here is to have the job applicant judged on the merits of actual productivity and not on the basis of assumed lack of productivity due to disability.

In practice, an employer's contact with market signals and indices of productivity will tend to be simultaneous, and an employer's concerns may have to be answered interchangeably. However, an employer's concern regarding the index of impairment can affect the assessment of productivity signals, which are the individual's job-skill indicators. Concerns about absenteeism, production quality, or need for supervision may stem from uncertain feelings about disability and may be unrelated to the individual in question. Both job-seekers and rehabilitation professionals need to recognize this distinction between how employers respond to market signals and how they respond to indices. Also at issue are job modification and architectural barrier removal, which can permit the skilled worker to be productive. Without such modifications, a person's productive skills may be inaccessible. The employer, lacking knowledge of modifications or fearing high modification costs, may tend to overestimate obstacles to the worker's productive capabilities.

It is important to note also that while an employer may have or develop a generally favorable attitude toward hiring persons with disabilities, the actual hiring may be delayed or avoided due to an uncertainty about exactly how to go about it. Furthermore, the employer may have real concerns about the costs and implications of hiring and the responses of supervisors and co-workers to the new employee. Employers may seek ways to work with rehabilitation agencies in hiring and upgrading jobs for people who have disabilities.

The Report of the Industry-Labor Council of the White House Conference on Handicapped Individuals (1977) discusses many of these issues. Potentially, employers may see more obstacles than actually exist. The rehabilitation professional can provide reassurance and expertise, meeting these needs and developing ways of working with employers and unions. Various awareness programs, such as the Texas Awareness Program, are currently being implemented to meet these needs. The Human Resources Center's Management Training Seminar, currently in development, is also a way of responding to employers' concerns about hiring and upgrading workers with impairments. Research will be directed toward understanding the dynamics of change, if any, that occur as a result of such training. These programs explore directions rehabilitation professionals can take in the job search when working with clients and ways of lowering the cost for employers of hiring persons with disabilities.

The strategy that can be developed to maximize the amount of information available to clients and counselors includes the following considerations:

1. Identification of job lead sources
2. Use of community resources that are made available through the development of appropriate channels of communication and information networks
3. Pursuit of information in appropriately selected labor markets
4. Identification of ways to influence employer search and hiring decision patterns

5. Use of client job-seeking skills and counselors job development skills to maximize the visibility of client productivity levels
6. Implementation of job modification and architectural barrier removal techniques

Development of a strategy that integrates these considerations is designed to achieve optimal placement, considering labor market conditions and productivity levels. This strategy will largely define an information-gathering process that will permit an individual to decide to accept a job that affords a proper investment return and an opportunity for career enhancement. Counselors and clients are mutually responsible for achieving appropriate placements.

Career Enhancement

The placement act occurs when a person accepts a job offer. From then on, a person's career is modified by the actual experience of working on that job. A person's entire career development, which began in the stage of productivity enrichment, is a process that continues while the person is a part of the labor force. The amount of monetary and nonmonetary income that a person receives during the course of a career is determined by factors that can enhance or detract from the career. The rehabilitation process cannot be expected to continue over a person's work life. However, it should contribute to the quality of a career by enriching a person's productivity to a point where the worker can realize a suitable return from participating in the labor force. The rehabilitation counselor should also attempt to work with a client to find a suitable placement in the primary labor market that affords a good opportunity for adequate monetary and nonmonetary income.

Career enhancement is the eventual target of all rehabilitation services. However, it receives special attention during the follow-up stage, which begins when the client accepts a job offer. Follow-up, as used here, refers to ongoing counselor and client contact after placement occurs. It also includes employer-oriented follow-up activities, which are equally important. Figure 4 presents an overview of the follow-up process. In the state/federal rehabilitation system, post-employment services would be included within the follow-up process. Case closure should not occur until the client and counselor are sure that there is a reasonable expectation of career enhancement. Rehabilitation service delivery should continue uninterrupted until this determination is made. The counselor and client should carefully make this assessment together. To make the various aspects of this assessment clear, a brief literature review follows.

The rehabilitation process can have a significant impact on placement by helping a client consider the qualities of the job offered. This review process should continue during the short-term follow-up that is within the scope of rehabilitation. By carefully performing this assessment with the client, a counselor should be able to teach the client what the relevant career enhancement factors are. The client can later reconsider these whenever a career decision needs to be made. The Seventh Institute on Rehabilitation Issues (1969) has described criteria for suitable placement:

1. Client and employer are satisfied
2. Client is maintaining adequate interpersonal relationships and acceptable behavior in the job environment
3. Occupation is consistent with the client's capacities and abilities
4. Client possesses acceptable skills to perform or continue the work satisfactorily
5. Employment and working conditions will not aggravate the client's disability in the job setting and will not jeopardize the health and safety of himself/herself or others
6. Wage and working conditions conform to state and federal statutory requirements

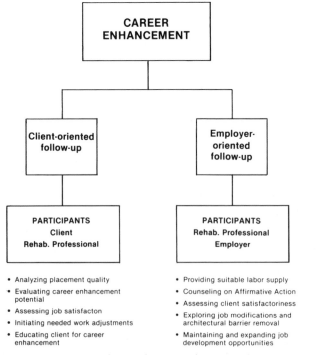

Figure 4.   Overview of selected processes in career enhancement.

7. Employment is regular and reasonably permanent
8. Client receives a wage commensurate with that paid other workers for similar work (p. 22).

To this list Dunn (1974) adds two additional considerations:

9. The job provides for upgrading and advancement within a reasonable period of time
10. The wage received is sufficient to enable the client and his family to obtain a minimally sufficient standard of living, as defined by the poverty level (p. 18).

It is evident that jobs providing these opportunities are in the primary labor market.

Lofquist and Dawis (1969) have presented a work adjustment model that addresses the variables that determine the tenure a person is likely to achieve on a given job. Basically, an interaction of four factors is involved. A person has certain *abilities* that must meet the *skill demands* of the job tasks. Also, a person has *needs* that must be met by the *rewards* offered by the job. If these four factors are congruent, tenure can be expected. This would imply that the person is satisfied with the job and also satisfactorily meets the demands of the employer. A dissatisfied worker might eventually quit whereas an unsatisfactory one might be fired. Instruments derived from this theory permit a counselor and client to anticipate the congruence between a client's skills and needs and a job's skill demands and rewards (Betz et al., 1966).

Herzberg (1966) has presented a theory based on worker needs that provides further insight into job maintenance. He presents a two-factor theory of needs. One factor relates to hygiene needs, which are similar to Maslow's lower order needs, such as physiological, security, and social needs. These needs are met by the environment. In particular, salary, working conditions, supervisor and co-worker, and company policies are important. Herzberg points out that if a job fulfills these needs, a worker will not be dissatisfied, but in order for a worker to become satisfied, additional needs must be met. Herzberg refers to these as motivator needs, which grow from a desire for personal fulfillment. These correspond to Maslow's higher order needs and are related to concepts of ego and self-actualization. These needs can be met only by the job content (i.e., what a worker actually does). The work itself; responsibility; and the availability of achievement, recognition, and advancement are critical elements in fulfilling motivator needs. Once these are met, a worker will be satisfied.

Issue has been taken with the exact theoretical picture of Herzberg's presentation, and the clear-cut distinction is probably artificial. However, his concepts have led to many efforts at job enlargement. These are attempts to increase motivator variables. This research has been used basically by employers who assume that job satisfaction is related to productivity. How workers might use these concepts to evaluate their career development and make decisions accordingly needs to be explored. Evidence suggests that work satisfaction is related to overall satisfaction with life (Friedlander, 1966). More research has to be conducted on this issue, but if the theory is substantiated, current efforts to expand the work roles of people who have severe disabilities is important. Systematic change must be pursued to enrich the jobs of persons with disabilities. Methods toward this end must be further developed and evaluated.

Herzberg's motivator variables are often linked to productivity. Since a person's productivity is directly related to labor force participation, a close look at other variables that correspond to productivity is necessary. Industrial psychologists have taken an extensive look at productivity. Korman (1971) has summarized much of this research. In brief, the motivation an individual has, the level of skill a person possesses, and the task and social requirements of the job combine to determine the productivity of the worker. All of these factors need to be considered by the client and counselor when evaluating a job offer and also when analyzing the suitability of a placement during the follow-up period.

Since rehabilitation services offered by any one program or agency can be active only over a brief time span during a person's career, the immediate follow-up period is important. The counselor and client must continue to evaluate the placement's career enhancement potential. This process must be structured so that the client can make an informed decision regarding a current job and can also learn how to use the same criteria in making other career enhancement decisions in the future. The counselor should probably not terminate follow-up until the client can independently make such an analysis.

If deficiencies in the current job indicate that career enhancement will be difficult, a new placement may be considered. However, the counselor and client should not overlook certain changes that could be initiated to alleviate the problems. Changes in client behavior, such as improved co-worker relationships, or in client routine, such as better transportation capability or personal hygiene, may adequately improve the situation. A client's productivity shortcomings might also be overcome by additional training or job coaching. Not to be overlooked are changes that can be initiated by the employer. Job modifications, barrier removal, and other reasonable accommodations may go far in helping to gain a productive and stable employee.

Up to this point in the discussion, follow-up has been presented as primarily an interaction between counselor and client. However, another central aspect of follow-up includes the interaction between counselor and employer. In this sense, the employer is also a consumer of rehabilitation services. The counselor can provide many meaningful services to employers that in the long run will benefit other rehabilitation clients. In the first place, regardless of future implications, the employer has expended funds in hiring the client. The counselor can help the employer realize a return on this investment by continuing to help the client maximize productivity during follow-up. Subsequent placement of job-ready clients will contribute to this process and also help the employer fulfill affirmative action requirements. If this can be accomplished, the employer will be more likely to pursue other activities that can benefit the counselor's service delivery. In this sense, follow-up activities can be viewed as job development. The counselor can include the employer in a new, informal communication network that will broaden the impact of rehabilitation services. The counselor can obtain valuable, local, world-of-work information from satisfied employers. Follow-up activities can provide data that can be used to influence what the counselor does with subsequent clients. Since all these benefits can proceed from employer-oriented follow-up activities, this aspect of the rehabilitation process needs appropriate attention.

This portion of the chapter has briefly outlined issues that affect job maintenance and career enhancement. The follow-up role of the counselor is to help a client determine the suitability of a placement, encourage and support client and employer changes to overcome problems, and teach the client how to independently monitor and change vocational circumstances that will maximize career enhancement. The counselor's follow-up activities must also attend to employer needs. If clients and employers can be adequately served during follow-up, the impact of rehabilitation services for subsequent clients can be greater. This will enhance the accomplishments and job satisfaction of the rehabilitation counselor. The importance of this effect should not be minimized.

REFERENCES

Becker, G. S. 1964. Human capital: A theoretical and empirical analysis, with special reference to education. National Bureau of Economic Research, New York.

Betz, E., Weiss, D. J., Davis, R. V., England, G. W., and Lofquist, L. H. 1966. Seven years of research on work adjustment. Minnesota Studies in Vocational Rehabilitation: Monograph 20. Industrial Relations Center, University of Minnesota.

Bowen, W. G., and Finnegan, T. A. 1969. The Economics of Labor Force Participation. Princeton University Press, Princeton.

Coleman, J. S., Katz, E., and Menzel, H. 1957. The diffusion of innovation among physicians. Sociometry 20:253–270.

Dunn, D. 1974. Placement services in the vocational rehabilitation program. University of Wisconsin-Stout, Research and Training Center. Menomonie, Wisconsin.

D'Zurrilla, T. J., and Goldfried, M. R. 1971. Problem solving and behavior modification. J. Psychol. 78:107–126.

Echols, F. H. 1972. Rehabilitation counselor's responsibility for placement. J. Appl. Rehab. Counsel. 3(2):72–75.

Ehrle, R. A. 1969. Rehabilitation counselor turnover: A review of the literature. Rehab. Counsel. Bull. 12(4):221–225.

Flannagan, R. 1974. Whatever happened to job placement? Voc. Guid. Quart. 22(3):209–213.

Freiman, M. P. 1976. Empirical tests of dual labor market theory and hedonic measures of occupational attainment. Unpublished doctoral dissertation, University of Wisconsin, Madison.

Friedlander, F. 1966. Importance of work and nonwork among socially and occupationally stratifed groups. J. Appl. Psychol. 5:437–441.

Granovetter, M. S. 1974. Getting A Job: A Study of Contacts and Careers. Harvard University Press, Cambridge.

Hart, W. R., and Karbott, M. J. 1964. Placement is counselor's job. Rehab. Rec. 5(1):1–10.

Heneman, H. G., and Yoder, D. 1965. Labor Economics. South-Western Publishing Company, Cincinnati, Ohio.

Herzberg, F. 1966. Work and the Nature of Man. New American Library, New York.

Hutchinson, J., and Cogan, F. 1974. Rehabilitation manpower specialist: A job description of placement personnel. J. Rehab. 40(2):31–33.

The Industry-Labor Council of the White House Conference on Handicapped Individuals. 1977. The report of the industry-labor council of the White House conference on handicapped individuals, handicapped workers and today's labor market. Washington, D.C.

Jaffe, A. J., Day, L. H., and Adams, W. 1964. Disabled Workers in the Labor Market. Bedminster Press, Totowa, New Jersey.

Jones, R. J., and Azrin, N. H. 1973. An experimental application of a social reinforcement approach to the problem of job finding. J. Appl. Behav. Anal. 6(3):345–353.

Kasper, H. 1967. The asking price of labor and the duration of unemployment. Rev. Econ. Stat. 49:165–172.

Katz, E. 1957. The two-step flow of communication: An up-to-date report on an hypotheses. Publ. Opinion Quart. 21:61–78.

Keith, R. D. 1976. A study of self-help employment seeking preparation and activity of vocational rehabilitation clients. Unpublished doctoral dissertation. Michigan State University, East Lansing.

Korman, A. K. 1971. Industrial and organizational psychology. Prentice-Hall, Inc., Englewood Cliffs, New Jersey.

Krippendorf, K. 1971. Communication and the genesis of structure. Gen. Syst. 16:171–185.

Lee, N. H. 1969. The Search for an Abortionist. The University of Chicago Press, Chicago.

Levitan, S. A., Mangum, G. L., and Marshall, R. 1972. Human Resources and Labor Markets: Labor and Manpower in the American Economy. Harper & Row Publishers, New York.

Lillehaugen, S. T. 1964. District placement counselors can boost jobs for handicapped. Rehab. Rec. 5(2):29–31.

Lippman, S. A., and McCall, J. J. 1976. The economics of job search: A survey. Econ. Inquiry 14:155–189.

Lofquist, L. H., and Dawis, R. V. 1969. Adjustment to Work—A Psychological View of Man's Problems in Work-Oriented Society. Appleton-Century-Crofts, New York.

McCall, J. J. 1970. Economics of information and job search. Quart. J. Econ. 84:113–126.

McClure, D. 1972. Placement through improvement of client's job-seeking skills. J. Appl. Rehab. Counsel. 3(3):188–196.

McDonald, D. J. 1974. The rehabilitation counselor: A resource person to industry, a revitalized approach to selective placement. J. Appl. Rehab. Counsel. 5(1):3–7.

Nagi, S. Z. 1977. Disability Policies and Programs: Issues and Options. Mershon Center, Ohio State University, Columbus, Ohio.

Nagi, S. Z., and Hadley, L. I., Jr. 1972. Disability behavior: Income change and motivation to work. Indust. Labor Rel. Rev. 25(2):223–233.

Perlman, R. 1969. Labor Theory. John Wiley & Sons, Inc., New York.

Rehabilitation Services Administration. 1977. Final report of characteristics in clients rehabilitation during fiscal year 1976. Information Memorandum, RSA-IM-77-71, Washington, D.C.

Salomone, P. 1971. A client-centered approach to job placement. Voc. Guid. Quart. 19(4):266–270.

Seventh Institute on Rehabilitation Issues. 1969. Recommended Standards for Closures for Cases. Rehabilitation Services Administration, Washington, D.C.

Sheppard, H. R., and Belitsky, A. H. 1966. The job hunt: Job seeking behavior of unemployed workers in a local economy. The W. E. Upjohn Institute for Employment Research. Johns Hopkins Press, Baltimore.

Spence, M. 1973. Job market signalling. Quart. J. Econ. 87:355–374.

Sussman, M. B., and Haug, M. R. 1970. From student to practitioner: Professionalization in rehabilitation counseling. Working Paper No. 7. Case Western Reserve University, Cleveland.

United States Bureau of the Census. 1972. Census of population, 1970, general social and economic characteristics, final report. PC (1) CIU.S Summary. U.S. Government Printing Office, Washington, D.C.

Usdane, W. M. 1974. Placement personnel—A graduate program concept. J. Rehab. 40(2):12–13.

Usdane, W. M. 1976. The placement process in the rehabilitation literature. Rehab. Lit. 37(6):162–167.

Whitten, E. B. 1975. The rehabilitation counselor, a historical overview. J. Appl. Rehab. Counsel. 6:55–59.

Wright, B. A. 1975. Social-psychological leads to enhance rehabilitation effectiveness. Rehab. Counsel. Bull. 18(4):214–223.

Zadny, J. J., and James, L. F. 1976. Another view on placement: State of the art, 1976. Regional Rehabilitation Research Institute, School of Social Work. Portland State University, Portland, Oregon.

Chapter 2

The Relationship of Vocational Evaluation and Vocational Placement Functions in Vocational Rehabilitation

Thomas W. Gannaway and William Wattenbarger

Editor's note: The authors continue a debate in this chapter that has been ongoing in rehabilitation for some time. The argument basically involves who is to do what within the rehabilitation process. This chapter reviews some of the traditional arguments concerning the roles and function of various rehabilitation professionals.

The authors also show how various role models have been derived from the existing service delivery system of the state/federal vocational rehabilitation system. The rationale for these models makes sense, but this chapter suggests that a functional review of the rehabilitation process indicates that a different set of role models can be established. This functional review is based on the use and flow of information in the delivery of rehabilitation services. Cases could be made for still other ways of organizing rehabilitation roles and functions, and research should be directed toward this. However, it is important to recognize the functional approach used in this chapter to analyze the rehabilitation process. This sort of functional analysis could be valuable in determining how rehabilitation programs are organized and administered.

The role models suggested in this chapter recognize the relevance of information to rehabilitation. Evaluation activities are reviewed with this in mind. Evaluation must provide data that permit an assessment of an individual in terms of the vocational implications of the information. Unless evaluation findings are relevant for the world-of-work context, vocational rehabilitation planning becomes a matter of trial and error. Vocational rehabilitation is in the business of providing services to enhance the vocational aspects of the lives of its clientele. Services offered within this context should be directed to this end.

A clarification of the relationship between vocational evaluation and placement can be approached in two ways. The usual approach is to review the existing literature and extrapolate to the current state of affairs. A review of the literature reveals little direct reference to the question of how vocational evaluation and placement are to relate. However the literature is extensive and largely of one mind regarding the intentions and functions of these two types of rehabilitation services (Dunn et al., 1974; Field et al., 1975; Zadny and James, 1976; Vandergoot and Jacobsen, 1978).

Sometimes it is more worthwhile to approach a subject with a fresh perspective. This approach can serve as a validity check on previous efforts and can give a new view of the subject. A fresh approach might eliminate confusion that may also exist in the development to date. This chapter approaches the problem of the relationship between vocational evaluation and placement from a more "classical philosophical" point of view, but also reflects pertinent literature. Certain assumptions about the profession of vocational rehabilitation (VR) are made, and the roles and functions of the various VR professionals are "deduced" from these assumptions.

VR PROCESS AND PROFESSIONAL ROLES

VR Process

The needs for expertise in several areas in VR have become evident. Among VR professionals today, one might include the vocational rehabilitation counselor (VRC), the vocational evaluator (VE), the vocational adjustment specialist, and the placement specialist. Each of these VR professions is working toward a definition of its unique roles and functions. The debate about the VRC's role and responsibilities has been continuing for decades and still much remains to be settled. The role and functions of the VE are also still being clarified. Both of these emerging professions form the basis for their own Division of the National Rehabilitation Association, they have their own literature, and they are moving toward the certification and licensure of their practitioners. Work adjustment and placement specialties are somewhat newer as VR professions than are VR counseling and evaluation. Nevertheless, much is being said about the need to professionalize these areas of VR service as well.[1] As recently as March, 1978, Field, Sink, and Gannaway (1978)

---

[1] Work adjustment is included in the same NRA Division with vocational evaluation, largely because these two functions have ordinarily been performed by the same professional or in the same facility. Placement has a division of its own. The professionalization of these two specialties is certainly well on its way. Still, the contention remains that these two are not as far advanced in this respect as are vocational evaluation and vocational rehabilitation counseling.

suggested the need to professionalize adjustment services in order to ensure quality service in that area. Lou Ortale spoke often of this pressing need (Ortale, undated). As early as 1964, Lillenhaugen (1964) was calling for a full-time placement specialty. Hutchinson and Cogan (1974) outlined a job description for a new professional they called the rehabilitation manpower specialist. Usdane (1976) presents a proposal for a master's level degree for placement specialists.

Some confusion remains regarding the overlap or interface between these professional roles. Some understanding of this confusion might be gained by looking again at what is called the rehabilitation process. Many diagrams of the VR process have been advanced, but the diagram in Figure 1 serves for the purposes of this exposition.

The numbers in the diagram are "case status" designations used in the state/federal VR programs representing a progression through phases of VR service delivery. The individual is first received and the initial background information collected. This information is reviewed and a determination made of what further evaluation or treatment is needed. Extensive evaluation of the person's skills, needs, interests, and work habits follows. Restoration and remedial services are selected and provided until the person is determined ready to work. The person is then placed in an appropriately selected job and monitored in this job until stability is achieved. Counseling and guidance are part of the process at all points.

The intuitive logic of such a conceptualization of the VR process is inescapable. This view clearly depicts what VR should be doing to help those it serves. It is suggested here that, in order to accommodate the diagrammed service responsibilities, the VRC has become conceptualized as the personification of the entire VR process. The VRC is seen as either doing it all or administrating the doing of it all by others. Cer-

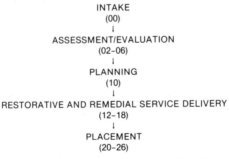

Figure 1.   Common representation of the VR process. The client receives the services sequentially, in principle. The numbers represent case status designations used in the state-federal VR programs.

tainly, a prominant view of the VRC is precisely this (McGowan and Porter, 1967; Whitehouse, 1974).

The primary criticism of such a view is that it is too much to ask of one person. Much of the continuing debate about the role and functions of the VRC centers on this point. No one person can possibly do all of the express and implied functions of the VR process, at least not well. The skills and knowledges throughout the VR process are energy and time consuming. No doubt is shed upon the intelligence and technical skills of practicing VR professionals to do any or all of these functions as needed. Rather, it is suggested that the constraint of time prohibits a single individual performing all these functions. If this is so, drastic reduction in case load size would be necessary to effectively deliver the full range of VR services in this manner.

Whatever criticism might be made of the VRC as the VR process personified, it is a holistic approach to human service delivery, and it does, in principle, afford a person a continuity of service and works against the dehumanization of the person served in many respects. There is much good in this holistic view and it should not be abandoned lightly.

While the personification of the VR process as one role may be conceptually simple and humanistic, it may be inefficient. The alternative is to specialize. Role models need to be created to meet the implied and express VR process functions. This logic is also inescapable, and it is this that largely accounts for the growing number of VR specialties. Not surprisingly, these specialties derive directly from the VR process model presented in Figure 1. Vocational evaluators are the embodiment of the evaluation phase. Work adjustment specialists are part of the treatment phase. Placement specialists have responsibility for the final phase of the process. In this context, the VRC assumes a more restricted role, providing the intake and data collection functions along with the coordination of specialized services and some counseling and guidance, but relieved of the placement and in-depth evaluative responsibilities.

The piecemeal personification of the VR process into specialties is not a totally satisfactory explanation of what has occurred. Some confusion (or overlap) remains between the functional domains of the respective professionals. Discussions of placement commonly dwell on evaluation and the determination of job readiness (an evaluation function) as preparatory to placement (Thomason and Barrett, 1960; Sinick, 1962). It is not uncommon to find placement issues discussed in the context of vocational evaluation processes (Pruitt and Pacinelli, 1969; Knape, 1972; Nadolsky, 1975).

One reason for the overlap in the discussions of role responsibilities may be the indivisible nature of the VR process. The phases are not really sequential steps as they appear to be. They are as likely to be simultaneous as not. A view of the VR process that leads to the definition of professional roles built upon sequential service delivery steps comes close but is unable to deal with situations in which a service from a "prior" or "subsequent" step is needed. For example, vocational guidance and work adjustment are both counseling functions, but typically the guidance occurs before and during evaluation whereas work adjustment follows evaluation in a facility. Vocational evaluation will sometimes evaluate a person's readiness for a given job by performing a job analysis as a standard by which to assess the person's skills, but there is no difference in the content of the job analysis done by an evaluator and one done by a placement specialist. The difference exists in why and when the analysis was done.

Some clarification may result if the element of timing is removed from the VR process model. An alternate VR process model is presented in Figure 2. Three kinds of things happen during the delivery of VR services: evaluation, counseling, and placement. The inevitable overlap with respect to when the types of functions occur remains. It is suggested that there are only three types of vocational rehabilitation functions, and the emphasis is on *vocational*. Of course medicine, orthotics and prosthetics, mental health counseling, and vocational education[2] are among the many rehabilitation specialties that are instrumental in the vocational rehabilitation of a person. They need not have a vocational intention, however. Healthy bodies, functioning limbs, and good mental health are valuable to have whether or not one intends to engage in productive activity resembling work. The three vocational rehabilitation professions devised from the evaluation, counseling, and placement functions are related by a unique set of three factors: a) a common client, b) a built-in interdependence of functioning, and c) the need to have an extensive and an intensive knowledge and understanding of the world of work.

It should be emphasized that the functions that translate into successful rehabilitation are relatively clear. It is the division of these functions among the various roles that is problematic. The role of a given VR professional is not immutable. The functions can be distributed in any number of ways. Which professional is to be responsible for which function will be determined by the size of the community, the nature of local business and industry, the availability of evaluation facilities, the state

---

[2] Vocational education is certainly a vocational service. It is not included in this discussion as a vocational rehabilitative profession because it is too specific, vocationally. Vocational education provides a client with a specific and perhaps narrowly applicable set of job skills. Vocational education does not require of its practitioners a broad (extensive and intensive) knowledge of the world of work. Each vocational educator must be skilled in a unique set of job skills. For this reason, the professional services of vocational education are seen here as "instrumental" for a client in much the same way that medical or orthotic services would be.

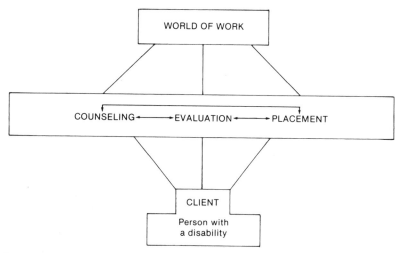

Figure 2.   The VR process conceived as three essential sets of functions that may occur simultaneously and that serve to facilitate the entry or reentry into the world of work of a person who has a disability.

and local structures for service delivery, the nature of the population served, and many other variables. Whatever distribution of functions is made, the VR process will remain functionally unchanged. Any attempt here to assign respective functions to roles would be of narrow applicability. In the following discussion emphasis is placed on the nature of evaluation and placement in particular as sets of functions that should be supported by the prevailing physical and administrative structures for service delivery.

Vocational Evaluation Functions

The goal of all VR services is to change things, whether in the person with a disability or in the environment, such that these persons can return to or enter the world of work, or at least have the opportunity to participate in the highest possible degree of independent living. Vocational evaluation purports to help achieve this goal through extensive assessment of each person's work potential through observation of behavior; through the determination of potential for training, restoration, or placement; and through helping to change behavior in order to upgrade employability and change self-concept (Bregman, 1967). Bregman points out correctly that this latter purpose is noticeably therapeutic in nature and falls more specifically in the realm of vocational counseling. Gellman (1968) summarized the vocational evaluation process as the observation, definition, and analysis of a person's work pattern, both from the perspective of personal attributes and from the perspective of demands likely to be made upon the person by the environment. This definition of vocational evaluation processes is rather neatly restricted to assessment functions.

A somewhat more contemporary statement of the objectives of vocational evaluation (Vocational Evaluation Services in the Human Services Delivery System, 1975) includes the identification of functional competencies and limitations, the determination of intervention strategies that will help to overcome the barriers to optimal outcome, and the provision of these services to eliminate a person's functional limitations where possible. Again, this latter function appears more precisely designated as a counseling function. Also in this report, a task force (Task Force #1) detailed the broad range of disability types, employment objectives, functionally disabling conditions, and service alternatives as they describe or pertain to the recipients of vocational evaluation services. In many respects vocational evaluation begins to assume many of the functional attributes, like that of the traditional VRC's role.

Vocational evaluation is perhaps better recognized by the tools or approaches utilized in assessment of individuals. Hoffman (1969) spoke of five "methodologies of work evaluation." He included job analysis, psychometric testing, work samples, the situational approach, work stations, and job tryouts. Nadolsky (1971) developed his model for the vocational evaluation of the disadvantaged in four sections, which he discussed as psychological testing, work sampling, situational approaches, and job tryouts. Task Force #2 (The Tools of Vocational Evaluation, 1975) conceived three types of tools associated with vocational evaluation: applied tools, situations as tools, and resource tools. The applied tools are those that involve the evaluator directly in the evaluation process, such as interviewing tools, observational tools, and recording/reporting tools. The situation tools are many but are represented in the broader classifications of on-the-job evaluation, work samples, and psychometrics. These tools are most uniquely identified with vocational evaluation. The resource tools are defined as information sources that serve to aid the evaluation process, including job analysis and occupational information, client information, and audiovisual materials. The Task Force #2 reports: "The uniqueness of vocational evaluation lies in its use of work-related activities and situations to assess human potential as it relates to the world of work."

Vocational evaluation then is a process of assessment of potential, especially with respect to an individual's optimum potential for vocational functioning, arrived at through a variety of sources, but characteristically through the observation of an individual's behavior in work-related or work-like activities. The omission of the direct provision of therapeutic services is deliberate. Certainly the practicing vocational evaluator is likely to be engaged in counseling and guidance, work adjustment, and even placement services as part of working with people in a given setting, but these services, although valuable, are not intrinsically evaluative functions.

Vocational Placement Functions

In most cases, the culminating service in the VR process would ideally be placement. The placement of a person with a disability is the traditional measure of the effectiveness of VR services. As noted in the introduction, much attention has been given to the importance of placement functions and a great deal of literature exists on placement issues. The functions commonly related to placement are outlined below.

Job Analysis   Job analysis is the process whereby a job is analyzed in terms of what demands it places upon the worker in that job. The variables upon which this analysis is made are conceivably as many as human creativity allows. Job analysis is typified by the extensive work done by the Department of Labor found in the *Dictionary of Occupational Titles* (1977). The process used to arrive at these job analyses is presented with some expansion in the *Handbook for Analyzing Jobs* (1972). One placement function then is the collection and utilization of job analysis information.

Occupational Information   Occupational information usually refers to all information about jobs (Baer and Roeber, 1964). In this chapter it refers to all job information that is not job analysis information. This would especially include information about the benefits that accrue to the worker in a given job, such as the salary scales, the advancement opportunity or career ladder, the contracted employee benefits, and the forecasted need for workers in each job. This definition admittedly runs somewhat counter to the usual definition of occupational information, but this liberty was taken because it was considered useful to maintain the distinction between the demands a job makes *of* the worker and the benefits that accrue *to* the worker. The collection and maintenance of local occupational information is also a placement function.

Job Development   Job development is the locating of possible specific job placements. The primary avenue through which this information is accumulated is employer contact and an understanding of employer hiring practices (Katz, 1957; Thomason and Barrett, 1960; Jones, 1966). Probably the most decisive factor in successful rehabilitation is the extent of information available about which jobs are open. Job development is a critical placement function.

Selective Placement   Selective placement is the process by which the needs and abilities of a person are matched with the job demands and need satisfiers implicit within a given job situation. This requires the ability to translate the findings of evaluation, if not provided in these terms, into the same terms as job analysis and occupational information in order to perform a good matching based on appropriate variables.

Job Engineering   In many cases, possible job placements are impeded by the particular limitations of a potential employee. In such cases these limitations might not prohibit the successful and satisfactory placement if the job, whether preexisting or new, is altered or created specifically to meet the needs of the person while still affording the employer the benefits of full productivity. The process by which jobs are constructed or modified to meet the specific needs of people is broadly referred to here as job engineering and includes the common notions of job modification and job restructuring.

Building Community Acceptance   The most subtle barrier to successful vocational rehabilitation is the prevailing community attitude regarding disability. Negative attitudes, apathy, and misunderstanding of the abilities of persons who have disabilities can make placement very difficult. A significant placement function in the VR process is to be involved with the community in an effort to change attitudes through the application of human relations, skills, and the education of the public with respect to the abilities of rehabilitated people. Employers and supervisors of workers (Sinick, 1968) are an important public target group in this regard.

The omission of evaluative and counseling functions as a part of placement is again obvious and intentional. From a specialization frame of reference, these are not placement functions.

The Relationship Between Evaluation and Placement Functions

Specialization is often attacked because it tends to be impersonal, i.e., a person is treated more as a subject matter than as a human being. Although impersonal service may be more likely to occur under specialized service delivery arrangements, this problem can be overcome with proper communication and sensitivity.

The probable source of this impersonalization is the difficulty encountered in attempting to maintain a continuity of service where many specialists are involved in service delivery. As discussed previously, the VR process is not a collection of neat and sequential episodes in a person's trek back from disability. Often the counseling, evaluation, and placement functions are performed simultaneously. The performance of any one type of function may depend upon the completion or initiation of another type of function. It is not unusual for a given VR professional to fill in for a colleague by providing more than one type of function when that colleague is not available. The solutions to these problems are largely administrative and legislative; however it is possible to speculate about the ideal arrangements under which the delivery of these three types of services can be optimized.

The Need for Communication Between Functions

The need for communication between functions is self-evident. The vital link between these sets of functions is the information derived by each, which should impact upon the others. Effective counseling must surely depend upon a complete evaluation of the person's needs and abilities and the nature of the demands to be encountered among the possible vocational objectives for that person. Evaluation can be performed with greater efficiency when complete initial information, including tentative vocational objectives and work history, is available. Evaluation also depends on the demand structures of job opportunities to guide truly useful recommendations for placement and the description of a person's vocational potential. A placement specialist cannot do an adequate job of selective placement unless the capabilities and needs of the person to be placed are known and expressed in terms that facilitate the matching of person and job attributes. These are but a few examples of the inescapable interdependence of these VR functions. The "stuff" that makes this interdependence work is information. The primary relationship among the evaluation, counseling, and placement functions is information sharing. These three functions, which were segregated in order to avoid overlap, must now be joined in order to provide complete VR services. Some intuitive ideas about communication of information might help in this task.

The combination of all these functions into one role has been claimed inadvisible, primarily due to time and caseload constraints, in the discussion of the traditional role of the VRC. This model, however, conceptually guarantees communication of relevant information between functions since all the information would have been obtained by a single professional.

Language Communication assumes language. It is suggested that the most appropriate language common to all phases of the VR process is the language of jobs, i.e., job analysis and occupational information, since all three types of functional VR processes are facilitated by a clear and extensive understanding of jobs. As it stands today, the language of job analysis is still primitive. Much improvement is needed in the extent and precision to which jobs can be described in measurable terms that will be useful to the counseling and evaluation efforts. The current factor/trait approach to job analysis found in the *Dictionary of Occupational Titles* (1977) is good, but neither final nor exclusive. The principle of job analysis is sound. The challenge to upgrade vocational language usage is clear for the VR professions.

Traditionally, evaluative information has been obtained from allied or related professionals, e.g., medical doctors, psychologists, educators, and social workers. This information is usually reported in a language and with a point of view especially suited to the purposes, needs, and traditions of the professional providing it. The translation of information received from these sources into terms having direct vocational significance is difficult and often faulty (Field and Wattenbarger, 1977). Nonetheless, the need to make this translation is unavoidable.

The importance of having a language about jobs that is common to all VR professionals involved in service delivery cannot be overemphasized. Such a language would help to facilitate a rapid, clear, and precise communication between professionals, and it would make matching individual qualifications and job demands no more difficult than it inherently is.

Means of Communication Having a common language is not enough. For communication to exist there must also be a medium to carry the information. The oldest and perhaps the most useful is the spoken word. Direct person-to-person communication of the information to be shared is at least timely. The conference table, the telephone, or across a desk are good opportunities to share pertinent information, when the allied professionals are available in this manner. To be available for direct personal communication of important service information, the representative professionals should be in the same building, such as a rehabilitation facility or office. Ideally each rehabilitation facility should have a placement specialist and a vocational counselor on the staff in addition to the vocational evaluator. These professionals would have responsibility for the functions discussed. This in-house team approach has the additional advantage of putting the respective professionals under one administration, which would greatly decrease the bureaucratic and administrative complication of cooperative effort. The discontinuity between functions is thus minimized.

Having the three sets of functions in different locations and under different administrations, i.e., in different agencies, is an inferior arrangement. The information and the person being served would have to travel much farther for the service to be delivered. The spontaneity of information-sharing and the ready clarification of information would be lost. The result would be the creation of "channels" through which the now largely written reports must flow. This could severely undercut the timely delivery of rehabilitation services.

The principle is simply this: the evaluation functions and the placement functions should be in as close a physical and administrative proximity as possible, and the direct spoken communication between these sources of information should be maintained as unencumbered by formal limitations as possible. The addition of the counseling function does not change this principle except to expand its application. There is certainly no escaping written reports as required records of intervention and assessment. Ongoing daily narrative reporting of information shared and received should serve much of this function while the formal reports are being prepared.

The notions of job banks (placement information) and skills banks (evaluation information) are no longer new. The idea is to match skills needed with skills available through some sort of matching system in order to effect a placement. The need for such a system has been suggested for many years (Bitter, 1968). Usually the systems have been manual, such as cards in files, folders in cabinets, or visual scan of microfiche listings of jobs from the Department of Labor Employment Service (Field, Grimes, and Decker, 1975). Recently new approaches to bringing an individual's abilities and job demands into closer compatibility have been tried with some notable success. Doane and Valente (1977) discussed a new role called job-coaching. Mallik and Sablowsky (1975) detailed how their "Job-Laboratory" worked and reported great success in placing the person judged unfeasible for rehabilitation. McCroskey et al. (1977) have devised and implemented a format that displays job analysis and individual evaluative information in juxtaposition for direct comparison.

The information impacting upon the delivery of rehabilitation services is voluminous. Manual processing of so much information is slow and imprecise because only a limited set of variables can be used to describe jobs and persons without confusion. The power of computers to handle great volumes of information and to manipulate or report this information is unquestioned. If access to the computer-based information banks were kept unencumbered, it would be possible to process many more variables per job/person and perform the matching function on this increased number of variables much faster. The output from the computer systems would have to be immediately available. Having to send away for information and then wait days or weeks is not likely to expedite services. The same principle applies here as before: the information is more useful and the services dependent upon the information more timely when the needed information is immediately and directly available to the individual receiving services and service providers.

Figure 3 shows the optimal relationship between the three sets of VR process functions diagrammatically. There must be a free flow of information between the three sets of functions. This is facilitated when all the information is reported in a common and precisely defined vocational language. The closest possible physical and administrative

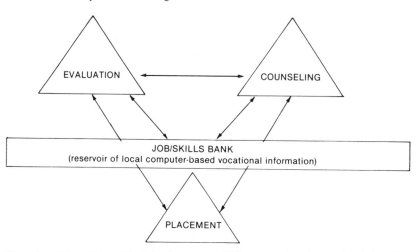

Figure 3.   Schematic model of the three types of VR process functions and their interface. Whereas placement almost always must transfer information by way of the bank to the other two functions, counseling and evaluation may use the bank to facilitate communication, but this is not necessary in every instance.

proximity between those professionals providing these services should be maintained. The vocational information should be directly and immediately available to individuals being served and professionals as needed. A vocational information library (job/skills bank), preferably computer based, including all possible job analyses and occupational information on a local basis, should be started and maintained.

The evaluation functions result in extensive analysis of an individual's vocational potential and service needs, which should be reported in "vocational language." These data are supplied to the job/skills computer bank once readiness has been determined and the person is jobseeking. The placement functions result in extensive analysis of the demands of jobs in the local area and the needs of local employers. These data, also in "vocational language," are supplied to the job/skills bank and maintained there even after placement has occurred in that job, to be used as resource information in the same manner as vocational information obtained from the *Dictionary of Occupational Titles*. The locally derived data will have greater utility because of its current nature and local specificity. The greatest utility of such a job/skills bank would be the rapid and exhaustive matching (selective placement) that would be possible with computer data processing.

REFERENCES

Baer, M. F., and Roeber, E. C. 1964. Occupational Information. Science Research Associates, Inc., Chicago.

Bitter, J. A. 1968. Toward a concept of job readiness. Rehab. Lit. 28(7):201–203.

Bregman, M. H. January 1967. The uses and misuse of vocational evaluation in the counseling process. *In* Some Recent Advances in Research in Vocational Evaluation. Research and Training Center in Vocational Rehabilitation, University of Pittsburgh, Pittsburgh, Pennsylvania.

Dictionary of Occupational Titles. 4th Ed. 1977. U.S. Department of Labor, Manpower Administration, Bureau of Employment Security.

Doane, R. C., and Valente, M. E. 1977. Role of job coaching in vocational rehabilitation. J. Rehab. 43(5):45–47.

Dunn, D. J., Currie, L., Minz, F., Scheinkman, N., and Andrew, J. 1974. Placement Services in the Vocational Rehabilitation Program. Research and Training Center, University of Wisconsin, Stout, Menomonie, Wisconsin.

Field, T. F., Decker, R., Grimes, J., and Watt, W. 1975. Bibliography on job placement (Job Placement Project). Unpublished manuscript, Rehabilitation Counselor Training Program, University of Georgia, Athens.

Field, T. F., Grimes, J. W., and Decker, R. S. August 1975. Abstracts of Local Projects (Job Placement Project). A collection of abstracted reports on local job placement approaches in Region IV, University of Georgia, Athens.

Field, T. F., Sink, J. M., and Gannaway, T. 1978. History and scope of adjustment services in rehabilitation. J. Rehab. 44(1):16–19.

Field, T. F., and Wattenbarger, W. 1977. Behavioral assessment format: Training Materials Manual, Rehabilitation Counselor Training Program. The University of Georgia, Athens.

Gellman, W. April 1968. The principles of vocational evaluation. Rehab. Lit. 29(4):98–106.

Handbook for Analyzing Jobs (Reprint 13). 1972. A manual developed by the U.S. Department of Labor, Manpower Administration. Available from the Materials Development Center, Stout Vocational Rehabilitation Institute, University of Wisconsin, Menomonie, Wisconsin.

Hoffman, P. R. 1969. Work evaluation: An overview. *In* W. A. Pruitt and R. N. Pacinelli (eds.), Work Evaluation in Rehabilitation (Reprint series RS-70-2). An educational guide developed from a conference held in Denver, Colorado. Available from the Materials Development Center, Stout State University, Menomonie, Wisconsin.

Hutchinson, J., and Cogan, F. 1974. Rehabilitation manpower specialist. J. Rehab. 40(2):31–33.

Jones, R. C. 1966. As you were saying—Selection and placement. (Abstract.) Personal J. 45(5):304–305.

Katz, E. 1957. The two-step of communication: An up-to-date report on hypothesis. (Abstract.) Public Opinion Quart. 21(Spring):61–78.

Knape, C. 1972. Placement: A try-out experiment. J. Rehab. 38(6):29–32.

Lillehaugen, S. T. 1964. District placement counselors can boost jobs for handicapped. Rehab. Rec. 5(2):29–31.

McCroskey, B. J., Wattenberger, W., Field, T. F., and Sink, J. M. 1977. Vocational Diagnosis and Assessment of Residual Employability Handbook. Published in limited edition. Available from the Rehabilitation Counselor Training Program, University of Georgia, Athens.

McGowan, J. F., and Porter, T. L. 1967. An Introduction to the Vocational Rehabilitation Process. Vocational Rehabilitation Administration, United States Department of Health, Education and Welfare.

Mallik, D., and Sablowsky, R. 1975. Model for placement-job laboratory approach. J. Rehab. 41(6):14–20.

Nadolsky, J. M. 1971. Development of a Model for Vocational Evaluation of the Disadvantaged. Auburn University, Auburn, Alabama.

Nadolsky, J. M. (Ed.). July 1975. Vocational Evaluation Project Final Report (Reprint No. 12). Originally published as three monographs, reprinted as a special edition of the Vocational Evaluation and Work Adjustment Bulletin. Available from the Materials Development Center, Stout State University, Menomonie, Wisconsin.

Ortale, L. The challenge of placement as a real professional service. Paper presented at a Placement Training Institute, Oklahoma State University. Available from the Clearing House, Rehabilitation Counselor Training Program, Oklahoma State University, Stillwater, Oklahoma. Undated.

Pruitt, W. A., and Pacinelli, R. N. (eds.). 1969. Work Evaluation in Rehabilitation (Reprint series RS-70-2). An educational guide developed from a conference held in Denver, Colorado. Available from the Materials Development Center, Stout State University, Menomonie, Wisconsin.

Sinick, D. August 1962. Placement training handbook. A training manual prepared with the aid of a Task Force coordinated by San Francisco State College and sponsored by the Office of Vocational Rehabilitation, U.S. Department of Health, Education and Welfare.

Sinick, D. 1968. Educate the community. J. Rehab. 34(3):25–27.

Thomason, B., and Barrett, A. M. September 1960. The placement Process in Vocational Rehabilitation. Vocational Rehabilitation Adminstration, U.S. Department of Health, Education and Welfare. (Reprinted November, 1964.)

The Tools of Vocational Evaluation. July 1975. A report of the Task Force #2. In J. M. Nadolsky (ed.), Vocational Evaluation Project Final Report (Reprint No. 12). Originally published as three monographs, reprinted as a special edition of the Vocational Evaluation and Work Adjustment Bulletin. Available from the Materials Development Center, Stout State University, Menomonie, Wisconsin.

Usdane, W. M. 1973. Placement—Process and professional training. Paper presented for the Lou Ortale Memorial Lecture, October 30, Atlantic City, New Jersey. Sponsored by the Job Placement Division, NRA, and the Lou Ortale Memorial Committee.

Usdane, W. M. 1976. The placement process in the rehabilitation of the severely handicapped. Rehab. Lit. 37:162–167.

Vandergoot, D., and Jacobsen, R. J. 1978. Annotated bibliography of placement-related literature. Unpublished paper, preliminary draft. Human Resources Center, Albertson, New York.

Vocational Evaluation Services in the Human Services Delivery System. July 1975. A report of the Task Force #1. In J. M. Nadolsky (ed.), Vocational Evaluation Project Final Report (Reprint No. 12). Originally published as three monographs, reprinted as a special edition of the Vocational Evaluation and Work Adjustment Bulletin. Available from the Materials Development Center, Stout State University, Menomonie, Wisconsin.

Whitehouse, F. A. 1974. The rehabilitation clinician: An emerging role. J. Rehab. 41(3):24–26.

Zadny, J. J., and James, L. F. 1976. Another view on placement State of the Art, 1976. (Abstract.) Studies in Placement Monograph No. 1, Portland, Oregon. Regional Rehabilitation Research Institute, School of Social Work, Portland State University, Portland, Oregon.

Chapter 3

Work Behavior Development and Placement

David B. Hershenson

Editor's note: Dr. Hershenson illustrates how concepts can be empirically researched, subsequently modified, and translated into applied activities in this chapter. He evolves practical counseling procedures from a conceptual view of how vocational development occurs.

The chapter suggests a counseling process that begins with a careful assessment of the individual client's stage of vocational development. It then proceeds to prescribe an intervention based on the assessment and indicates the type of outcome that counseling should lead to. It is important to recognize that this counseling process intends to link psychological concepts directly with world-of-work factors through a counseling process that uses a language consistent with both. As the previous chapter points out, this is an important development for the field of rehabilitation. A consistent terminology which integrates the various vocational rehabilitation activities from initial evaluation to long-term placement follow-up is offered here. Of course, other language systems are also possible. This model should be an example leading to further development in this area.

The system described here also indicates how work readiness might be defined in terms of vocational/psychological concepts. This would help clarify the relationship between placement specialists and rehabilitation counselors, should this arrangement be desirable. Using a standardized conceptual framework and language, counselors and placement specialists would be able to share each other's information more easily. Again, the importance of information within the rehabilitation process brings up the need to evaluate the reliability and validity of the information flowing among specialists.

Like most emerging areas of concern in rehabilitation, the topic of job placement is rife with controversies involving both the relative efficacy of different placement techniques and competing theoretical models for the placement process itself. For example, Salomone and Usdane (1977) have debated the issue of whether counselors should assist people with disabilities to develop their own self-placement skills or whether counselors should actively intervene in placement on their behalf. Most of the existing controversies concerning placement are spurious. The real question to be answered is *under what conditions* a given placement technique or theory is the right one. Based upon the line of research concerning vocational development reviewed in this chapter, a proposal is offered that states that the appropriateness of a given placement strategy or tactic depends upon the level of development of work-relevant behaviors on the part of the person to be served. Thus, a person with a poor self-concept as a worker, little work motivation, and no career goals requires a different sort of placement assistance than does a self-confident, highly motivated, goal-directed person. While this point may seem obvious, it has never been proposed as a coherent, testable model for the placement process. This chapter proposes such a model. It is, moreover, the intention of the author that this model be one that can be used effectively by placement specialists who lack extensive counseling skills.

BACKGROUND: LIFE-STAGE
VOCATIONAL/WORK BEHAVIOR DEVELOPMENT

Hershenson (1968a) suggested that vocational development could be conceptualized as a five-stage, sequential process. These stages, defined by the way a person uses energy, are: 1) Social-Amniotic (energy used for awareness), 2) Self-differentiation (energy used for control), 3) Competency (energy is directed), 4) Independence (energy becomes goal-directed), and 5) Commitment (energy is invested). Each stage addresses a specific vocational question: 1) Am I? 2) Who am I? 3) What can I do? 4) What will I do? and 5) What meaning does what I do have for me? Consequently, each requires a different measurement construct: 1) Socialization, 2) Self-concept, attitudes, and values, 3) Abilities, 4) Interests, and 5) Satisfaction.

In a subsequent series of studies, Hershenson and his colleagues tested the proposition that the last four of these stages were sequential in development. The first stage, Social-Amniotic, which involves vocationally relevant background factors, was excluded because it represented diffuse, idiosyncratic environmental variables that could not be consistently related to specific intrapsychic phenomena. Therefore, Hershenson et al. hypothesized that individuals would score higher on measures of early intrapsychic stages than on measures of the subsequent ones: that is, individuals would score highest on Self-differentiation, which involves self-concept as a worker and work motivation; next highest on Competence, that is, work habits, work skills, and work-related interpersonal relations; next on Independence, the appropriateness and crystallization of vocational goals; and lowest on Commitment, the person's satisfaction and satisfactoriness in an occupation.

Hershenson and Langbauer (1973), using a sample of 222 deaf persons in a rehabilitation program who were divided into four groups (high and low functioning workshop and counseling groups), found that in all groups, average Self-differentiation ratings exceeded average Competence ratings, which in turn exceeded average Independence ratings. The ratings on Commitment did not consistently conform to the predicted sequence, but it was recognized that this category, like Social-Amniotic, involved factors external to the subject. For example, satisfactoriness is determined by a supervisor's rating and hence was not purely intrapsychic. Thus, the predictions concerning the sequence of ratings on the three purely intrapsychic stages of vocational development (Self-differentiation > Competence > Independence) were supported. This same sequence of intrapsychic stages was found in a sample of 314 inner-city, socially disadvantaged Model Cities project clients and in a sample of 90 mid-career changers (Hershenson and Lavery, 1978). Different rating formats were used in all three studies. The first two studies used ratings by counselors, while the mid-career changers did self-ratings. The three studies used persons with disabilities and poverty-level and middle class subjects, thus covering a broad spectrum of individuals. The consistent findings in these three studies over a wide range of subjects and measurement techniques support the original proposition about the sequential nature of the three intrapsychic stages.

In addition to postulating and demonstrating the existence and sequence of these stages, Hershenson (1969) also suggested that each transition from one stage to the next required a different type of counseling intervention, depending on the particular stage of development of the person and the severity of the difficulty the person was having in making the transition. Thus, the transition from Self-differentiation to Competence required information input. The transition from Competence to Independence required information processing, and the transition from Independence to Commitment required information utilization. Depending on the severity of the problem, the counselor's function in any transition might be facilitation, which involves promoting normal development in the absence of severe problems or remediation, that is, actively removing serious blocks to normal development.

This theoretical model for assistance techniques was applied to sheltered workshop practices (Hershenson, 1968b), and appeared to have heuristic value. Some empirical support for the postulated use of different techniques for dealing with different transitional issues was provided by a study reported in Melhus, Hershenson, and Vermillion (1973). These researchers found that high school students who scored low on a measure of academic and personal coping ability improved more on a measure of appropriateness of occupational choice when given personal counseling than when given access to an interactive, computerized, vocational information system. Students who scored high on the measure of academic and personal coping ability, however, improved equally regardless of which treatment was employed.

From this line of theoretical and empirical studies, it seems appropriate to come to three conclusions. First, the intrapsychic process of vocational development involves three stages: Self-differentiation, Competence, and Independence. Second, these stages develop sequentially. Finally, different types of counseling intervention are differentially effective at each stage, depending on the nature and severity of the developmental issue involved.

In a more recent publication, Hershenson (1974) extrapolated these findings to the more general concept of work behavior. In doing so, the constituent elements of the three stages were retained, but the names of the stages were changed. Thus, "Self-differentiation" was changed to "Work Personality" but retained the components of self-concept as a worker and work motivation. "Competence" was changed to "Work Competencies" but retained the components of work habits, work skills, and interpersonal relations in the work setting. Finally, "Independence" was changed to "Work Choice" but retained the components of appropriateness and crystallization of vocational goals. Hershenson recognized that although these three stages develop sequentially, they have an interactive feedback effect on each other. Thus, Work Personality develops before Work Competencies, but when Work Competencies do develop, they in turn have an impact on Work Personality. For example, one need only observe the effects of learning disabilities on the self-concepts of school children.

THE MODEL: WORK
BEHAVIOR DEVELOPMENT AND PLACEMENT

To apply the three-stage model of work behavior development to the placement process, one must integrate an intrapsychic process with a reality-based process, control of which is in large measure external to the individual, as in the case of the labor market. Nonetheless, based on the material presented previously, a model for the placement process can be proposed. In this model, the phases and the elements within each phase are sequential. Each phase and element within it presupposes the substantial accomplishment of the prior phases and elements; however, the existence of interactive feedback is also recognized.

Phase I.   Pre-placement exploration (self-awareness). This stage involves *information input*. It utilizes the intrapsychic elements of:
   A.   Work Personality
   B.   Work Competencies
        Once the client has a relatively clear conception of his:
        1.   self-concept as a worker
        2.   work motivations
        3.   work habits (e.g., punctuality, neatness)
        4.   work skills (including functional capacities)
        5.   interpersonal skills in the work setting
        one can move to:

Phase II.   Placement understanding (job awareness). This stage involves *information processing*. It utilizes:
   A.   The intrapsychic element of Work Choice
   B.   The externally based element of the client's knowledge of jobs
        Once a client has a relatively clear conception of:
        1.   the appropriateness of the client's work goals
        2.   the crystallization of these work goals
        3.   the existence of jobs in the economy that conform to these goals
        one can move to:

Phase III. Placement action (job search skills). This stage involves *information utilization*. It utilizes the externally based elements of:
   A.   Locating an appropriate job
   B.   Attaining that job
        It requires the client to have a clear conception of:
        1.   job-hunting techniques
        2.   job-landing techniques

Finally, it is postulated that the role of the counselor (or placement specialist, as the case may be) is:

            a.   to determine where in this sequence the client is functioning (e.g., does the client have good self-awareness concerning his work personality and work competencies?)

b. to determine the severity of the problem at the element at which the person is experiencing difficulty (e.g., if the client lacks clear self-awareness about work motivation, is this due to inability to integrate understanding already available or is this due to a paucity of relevant experiences from which to gain understanding?)

c. based on the severity of the deficit, to undertake an appropriate program of facilitation (for relatively minor impediments) or of remediation (for major impediments)

d. once the deficit is overcome, to help the client move through the remaining phases of the placement process, culminating in successful placement in a job that the client is capable of performing, retaining, and enjoying

This sequence of phases in the placement process is spelled out in Table 1.

Table 1 also indicates procedures the placement counselor might use to assist a person at any given level of development (phase and element within it) or level of severity of problem. This would involve facilitation for mild problems, remediation for severe ones. Thus, if the counselor/placement specialist determines that some people are somewhat uncertain about their self-concepts as workers or their work motivation, but they have had experiences that would help sort these matters out, then the counselor might assist them by using a facilitative technique such as values clarification. If, however, the counselor determines that their work personalities (i.e., self-concepts as workers and/or work motivation) are in disarray and that they lack the internal resources or experiences from which to draw in sorting these issues out, then the counselor must employ a remediational technique, such as referring them to a therapeutic workshop. There, these individuals can confront and work out the difficulties they have in establishing work personalities.

Pre-placement Exploration

According to the model proposed in this chapter, the counselor must first evaluate and, where necessary, provide appropriate assistance to people on the issue of their work personalities. When the counselor evaluates work personality as being well established, that is, when the counselor sees a clear, positive self-concept as a worker and a strong work motiva-

Table 1. Phases in the placement process

Phase	Aim	Elements	Counselor assistive procedures	
			Facilitation	Remediation
Pre-placement exploration (information input)	Self-awareness	Work Personality[a] Self-concept as a worker Work motivation	Values clarification	Therapeutic workshop
		Work Competencies[a] Work habits Work skills Interpersonal skills at work	Identify assets	Prevocational training
Placement understanding (information processing)	Job awareness	Work Choice[a] Appropriateness of goals Crystallization of goals	Nondirective examination	Directive guidance
		Identification of jobs conforming to work choice[b]	Use of occupational information	Transitional or trial employment
Placement action (information utilization)	Job search skills	Job-hunting techniques[b]	Organizing job hunt; résumé writing	Job development
		Job-landing techniques[b]	Handling applications and interviews	Selective placement

[a] Intrapsychic.
[b] External.

tion, either from the time that the person enters the placement process or as a result of an assistive procedure instituted by the counselor, the issue of work competencies arises. If the counselor evaluates work habits, work skills and functional capacities, and work interpersonal relations as being strong and clear to the client, then the counselor may move the placement process into the next phase. If, however, the counselor finds that work competencies are present but unclear to the person, then a facilitative assistance procedure such as working with the person to identify assets is called for (see Anthony, Pierce, and Cohen, 1977). This procedure presupposes that the person has had experiences, such as successful work or school performances, from which work competencies may be identified. Sometimes work competencies and positive experiences from which these strengths may be understood are lacking. In that case, the counselor must provide these experiences and resultant work competencies through such remediational procedures as prevocational training for the development of work habits and work-related interpersonal skills and/or skills training for the development of work skills. The counselor should not begin to work with issues of work competencies until issues of work personality are fairly well resolved. Conversely, when the counselor determines that the person has pretty well resolved the issues of both work personality and work competencies, the pre-placement exploration phase is complete, and the counselor is ready to move with the person to the second phase, placement understanding.

Placement Understanding

The second phase, placement understanding, also has two sequential elements: work choice and job identification. Work choice presupposes the successful resolution of problems with work personality and work competencies. For the person whose work choice is both appropriate and crystallized, no intervention is necessary. For the person who is uncertain about work choice, a facilitative procedure, such as nondirective examination, should serve to help formulate a choice well matched to the person's work personality and work competencies. For the person whose work choice is very unclear or conflicted, a remediational procedure, such as directive guidance, may be called for. In this process, the counselor may help direct the person toward a choice that is suitable to work personality and work competencies. It may be noted that the distinction between facilitative, nondirective examination and remediational, directive guidance lies in how active a role the counselor must assume in interpreting the conclusions arrived at during the pre-placement exploration phase and the implications these conclusions have for the person's work choice. Thus, one is really speaking of a continuum of active intervention by the counselor. Insofar as is possible, the process should be client-centered so that the work choice arrived at is one that the person can "own." The more the counselor dominates the process, the greater the risk that the person will reject the outcome.

Once the person has arrived at a work choice, the intrapsychic part of the placement process is over; that is, one moves from the personal view of self to the need to come to terms with external realities. It is posited, however, that unless persons have first gained a coherent understanding of their work personalities, work competencies, and work choices, they cannot effectively understand the job market or become involved with the process of searching for a job.

The second element in the placement understanding phase is the identification of jobs that are consistent with the person's work choice. For some people, the work choice may point directly to a specific job. Indeed, the two may be synonymous. However, for others, the work choice may represent a more diffuse area, defined by a desire, such as "helping people" or "working on engines." Should a person require some help with identifying jobs in a specific area, the use of occupational information may be a facilitative procedure. Should a person, however, be very unsure of how to translate a desirable kind of work to a specific job, then transitional or trial employment may be used as a remediational procedure. The "hands on" nature of such activity may both test and bring into focus possible job alternatives. Once a job (or range of choices) that corresponds to the overall work choice has been identified, the second phase of the placement process, placement understanding, is complete and the person is ready for the third phase, placement action. This phase essentially involves the implementation of job-search skills.

Placement Action

Placement action involves the development and use of job-hunting and of job-landing techniques. For people who are capable of finding and landing their own jobs, facilitative procedures such as organizing a job hunt or preparing a résumé will teach them to find jobs. To land a job, skills such as knowing how to handle job application forms, role playing, and job interviews are appropriate. For the person who requires intervention by the counselor, that is, a person with minimal skills and/or a severe disability, the counselor must assume a more advocacy-oriented role, undertaking the remediational procedures of job development and selective placement.

SUMMARY

This chapter has suggested that placement may be considered as a three-phase process: pre-placement evaluation (to provide information input), placement understanding (to allow information processing), and placement action (to implement the information gained and decisions made in the two prior phases). These phases each have two elements. First, work personality and work competencies must be defined, which will in turn permit a work choice that can be related to existing jobs. Then the person can be assisted in locating and landing one of these jobs. These six elements are sequential in nature.

It is the job of the placement counselor to evaluate the clients' achievement of each successive element. Based on the evaluation, the counselor may conclude that a client has achieved an element and needs no help, that the client needs some assistance in the form of "facilitation," or that major intervention ("remediation") is needed to achieve that element and thus move on to the next one.

The process discussed in this chapter only carries the counselee-counselor relationship up to the point of job placement. This is not meant to imply that the counselee-counselor relationship should end at that point. Follow-up counseling after placement for job maintenance and evaluation are clearly necessary.

The model presented here offers a number of interesting research questions, such as the accuracy of ordering the last three elements. The first three elements were presented in an empirically validated sequence, but the last three are in a logically derived sequence. Hence they require empirical validation. It may well be that these last three elements involve interactive feedback with each other and with the first three elements as well. For example, a person who develops excellent job-hunting techniques may find that none of the jobs identified in the prior phase is available. This may lead to a need to identify other, somewhat related jobs or even to reassess the work choice. This in turn may lead to a need to review work competencies. Thus the counselor may have to move back one or more steps in the sequence and start the process again if insurmountable obstacles should arise. Other research questions relate to the efficacy of the suggested procedures for facilitation and remediation and to defining operationally the point at which a person's developmental blockage at a given element is severe enough to require remediation rather than facilitation.

The purpose of this chapter has been to present a model for the placement process that takes into account both a person's internal level of work behavior development and the external realities of finding a job. It has been suggested that preparing for placement must be conceived of as a sequential process rather than as a single act. The phases and constituent elements that comprise that process have been suggested, together with techniques to assist a person in achieving each element. It is the writer's hope that this model will both help systematize counseling for the placement process and generate research concerning the specific efficacy of various placement techniques.

REFERENCES

Anthony, W. B., Pierce, R. M., and Cohen, B. F. 1977. Psychiatric rehabilitation practice: The skills of career placement. Book 5. (Draft Copy). Carkhuff Institute of Human Technology, Inc. Cited with permission of first author.

Hershenson, D. B. 1968a. Life stage vocational development system. J. Counsel. Psychol. 15:23–30.

Hershenson, D. B. 1968b. A vocational life stage approach to sheltered workshop practice. J. Rehab. 34:26–27.

Hershenson, D. B. 1969. Assisting life stage vocational development. Person. Guid. J. 47:776–780.

Hershenson, D. B. 1974. Vocational guidance and the handicapped. *In* E. Herr (ed.), Vocational Guidance and Human Development, Chapter 19. Houghton Mifflin Co., Boston.

Hershenson, D. B., and Langbauer, W. R. 1973. Sequencing of intrapsychic stages of vocational development. J. Counsel. Psychol. 20:519–521.

Hershenson, D. B., and Lavery, G. J. 1978. Sequencing of vocational development stages: Further studies. J. Voc. Behav. 12:102–108.

Melhus, G. E., Hershenson, D. B., and Vermillion, M. E. 1973. Computer assisted vocational choice compared with traditional vocational counseling. J. Voc. Behav. 3:137–144.

Salomone, P. R., and Usdane, W. M. 1977. Client-centered placement revisited: A dialogue on placement philosophy. Rehab. Counsel. Bull. 21:85–91.

Chapter 4

Planning for Job Placement

Jerry J. Zadny

Editor's note: Both counselors and administrators will profit from reading this chapter. Dr. Zadny points out that structured planning for placement will enable a job-seeker to begin successful career development. Counselors and job-seekers can, by using placement plans, take a realistic look at the training needs of the job-seeker and evaluate the disincentives to successful job placement.

A realistic evaluation of the skills and needs of a job-seeker can eliminate waste and inefficiency in the rehabilitation process. Counselors need not waste time teaching job preparation skills in areas in which the job-seeker is already well prepared. Similarly, job-seekers need not be burdened with training and preparation for jobs that do not offer remuneration sufficient to offset the loss of benefits from Social Security, Disability Insurance, and Medicare.

Evidence shows that counselors who plan for placement have higher success rates than those who do not. In addition, the author points out that counselors who prepare placement plans distinct from the Individualized Written Rehabilitation Plan have more placements. This may result from the application of more counselor time to the placement plan, but the author is cautious in his claims because causality is tenuous.

Finally, the author provides a sample placement plan that counselors can use as a basis for developing sophisticated placement strategies.

The capacity to mobilize and coordinate diverse services to achieve a clearly defined goal has distinguished client services in the federal/state rehabilitation program from those in other human service agencies. No other program can claim as wide a range of resources, as definite a goal as job placement, or as impressive a record of effectiveness. Planning of the kind reflected in the Individualized Written Rehabilitation Plan (IWRP) required by legislative mandate and developed for each client has been a key to that success. Extension of the planning process to placement and the steps necessary to find a job may be an important vehicle for making further progress.

In developing rehabilitation plans, counselors often concentrate on increasing a person's potential for productive work to the extent of ignoring the ultimate problem of finding a job. Restoration and training usually precede placement, but concentrating on them exclusively confuses means with ends. Building competence does not ensure employment. The skills required to hold a job are different from those necessary to find one. The kinds of assistance a counselor provides in helping a person prepare for work and a career are different from those provided for job search. Planning for placement is a way to assure that prior enrichment of a person's potential for work will be realized in a successful career, regardless of a disability.

Placement technique has developed beyond the point of simply matching a person with a job slot or selling an employer on a person's abilities. Labor market forecasts can be used to select promising occupations and to avoid unpromising ones. When appropriate, job analysis and job modification can be applied to identify and create new openings. Many persons profit from instruction in job-seeking skills. The availability of post-employment services gives counselors the latitude to go further than before to assure an adequate adjustment to work and to go beyond simply finding a job to address issues of career development. None of these functions can be performed effectively unless it is carefully integrated with other services.

Increased service to persons with severe disabilities makes placement planning all the more essential. Severe disability not only limits the range of occupations available and heightens employer resistance, but it also increases the level of compensation a person must seek to offset the loss of existing income and medical benefits upon becoming employed. If these realities are not dealt with, persons will be prepared for jobs they will not be able to obtain or cannot afford to accept. For persons entering the labor market for the first time or embarking on a new occupation, a good placement is more than just a job, it is the beginning of a career. Job mobility is a particular concern for persons with disabilities, since entry level positions can often become dead ends. The next higher position may not accommodate the person's disability, or the person may not be aware that many workers change firms to advance. Planning that anticipates a career ladder avoids pigeonholing persons in jobs with no future and thereby allows them to realize their potential.

The notion of developing a placement plan is not new. The practice is recommended in the report of the Ninth Institute on Rehabilitation Services (1971, p. 13). What is new is the pressure counselors in state agencies are experiencing to serve more difficult cases than ever before and, consequently, to make use of the best placement techniques available. One way of responding to that pressure is for counselors to implement placement planning.

The results of a survey of 208 counselors in seven western states which tied reported placement practices to performance in getting people jobs indicate that although planning is not the rule, counselors who do plan enjoy a higher success rate (Zadny and James, 1977). The counselors, who represented a random sample of state agency staff, were asked to recount how extensively they cover placement in the IWRPs they write, whether they are required to incorporate a distinct placement plan in the IWRP, and whether they are required to write a placement plan separate from the IWRP. Table 1 displays the percentages of counselors who reported customarily including each of nine placement-related elements in rehabilitation plans they write. Coverage of placement was less than comprehensive. For example, only 27% of the counselors note the level of compensation to be sought and less than half record potential sources of job leads. Not many of us would embark on training for a new

Table 1.   Coverage of placement in IWRPs

	Percent yes
Which of the elements listed are commonly recorded in the general plan you write for job seekers:[a]	
Indication of level of compensation sought	27
Potential sources of job leads	38
Steps for training in job-seeking skills	45
Likely problems job-seekers will encounter in seeking work	61
Allotment of specific responsibilities to job-seeker and counselor	71
A timetable for locating leads, filing applications	14
Notation of how post-employment follow-up will proceed	40
Statement of probable post-employment assistance or adjustment services required	47
Specification of services and assistance required by job seeker to seek work	52

[a] First five elements are associated with more rehabilitations in general, and also with those having severe disabilities.

Table 2. Placement plans, rehabilitations, and percentage of cases closed as not rehabilitated

	Total number of successful rehabilitations in 1 year	Percentage of cases closed as not rehabilitated
Does your office policy require that a plan for placement be incorporated in the general plan?		
Yes N = 132	29.4	25
No N = 76	26.5	24
	$t = 1.10$; not significant	$t = 0.18$; not significant
Does your office policy require that a plan for placement be written separately?		
Yes N = 39	36.1	18
No N = 169	26.6	26
	$t = 2.24$; $p < 0.01$	$t = 2.94$; $p < 0.01$

career without some idea of what the pay will be or of the prospects of obtaining a job, yet this seems to be what many persons are asked to do by their rehabilitation counselors when their IWRPs omit such information. Correlations between the elements reported as included in plans and placement rates were not significant, but inclusion of the first five items in the table in IWRPs was uniformly associated with obtaining more rehabilitations and more rehabilitations of persons with severe disabilities.

It can be argued that it is premature to consider the details of placement at the outset of rehabilitation because circumstances change over the time it takes to complete an average program. If this is so, it would be more appropriate to cover the steps necessary to secure a job later in a separate plan when the person is approaching placement. The data summarized in Table 2 support this reasoning. When counselors were asked whether their agencies required that they discuss placement in the general plans they write, there was no appreciable difference in placement rates for those reporting the requirement and those not. In contrast, counselors who indicated that they are required to write a separate placement plan had 35% more rehabilitations and a 31% lower incidence of cases closed as not rehabilitated than other counselors. The correlational nature of the research precludes casual interpretation, but the implication is that planning mediated the superior outcomes.

Poor employer reception and poor motivation on the part of the job-seeker are often cited by counselors as being significant obstacles to placement (Thoreson et al., 1968; Zadny and James, in press). In the survey, counselors were asked to name the three most serious problems encountered by their clients as they look for work. Those who reported that they are not required to write a separate placement plan were five times as likely to cite poor employer reception of applicants as being a problem and half again as likely to mention the job-seekers' lack of motivation to work or to seek work than those required to write separate plans. Again, planning appears to be related to better placement outcomes. In this case, it may alleviate some of the unpleasantness associated with job search by helping persons overcome employer resistance and by bolstering the person's ability to persevere.

Looking for work is aversive. Planning may be one way of making the process a little less painful.

ELEMENTS OF SOUND PLANNING

The goal of placement planning is to secure a good job at a fair wage. This entails anticipating and resolving potential problems before they occur, teaching people to describe their skills advantageously, and limiting the inconvenience and stress associated with job search by recommending effective methods. A person must be able to locate potential employers through counselors and other sources and to obtain job offers.

Planning need be no more complex than the problems a particular client faces. The basic elements are:

1. An assessment of the need for training in job-seeking skills
2. The wage and other compensation necessary to maintain a person's standard of living and to offset loss of existing benefits
3. A list of potential sources of job leads that capitalizes on the proven effectiveness of informal sources, such as family and friends
4. Assignment of respective counselor and job-seeker responsibilities
5. Anticipated post-employment services
6. A reasonable timetable for locating openings, for filing and following up on applications, and for checking progress

The purpose of each element is for the most part self-evident, but some warrant special comment.

The importance of attending to job-seeking skills is hard to over-emphasize. Hiring decisions are only partially influenced by ability.

Hamilton and Roessner's (1972) study of 280 employers of WIN program graduates found that non–job-related characteristics were given at least as much weight in hiring as the applicant's job-related abilities. For example, good personal appearance was more likely to be a required qualification (75%) than either specific training (28%) or specific experience (23%). Experimentation with instruction in job-seeking skills has consistently demonstrated the effectiveness of such programs. McClure (1972) reported that 50% of the participants in a group-administered class were employed within 30 days, as opposed to 24% of the subjects in a comparison group who were not given the training. Keith, Engelkes, and Winborn (1977) cite employment rates of trained and untrained subjects to be 42% and 10%, respectively, after 2 months following a program based on individual instruction. Because subjects were randomly assigned to experimental and control groups in each instance, the subjects' job-related skills were not at issue. The subjects who received the training were more successful because they were better prepared to convince employers to hire them.

The hiring process often involves a series of decisions on the part of the employer, including a screening based on written applications, an interview, and subsequent decision by personnel to refer or not refer an applicant to the department with an opening, and final disposition by the person responsible for supervising the vacant position. To get a job, the job-seeker and the counselor must influence each decision in the job-seeker's favor. Preparation in job-seeking skills can help a person describe personal abilities favorably, convey enthusiasm about the job, and explain why disability will not interfere with productivity.

Setting a target wage identifies disincentives before the job-seeker and counselor waste time on jobs that cannot pay enough to maintain a reasonable standard of living. Listing likely sources of job leads starts the person on the right track. Studies of job-finding among persons with a disability suggest that patterns are not markedly different from those of workers without disabilities (Jaffe, Day, and Adams, 1964: Veglahn, 1975; Zadny and James, 1978). Conventional sources such as the want ads, state employment service, and private agencies are used at rates far in excess of any justified by their likelihood of paying off. Informal sources, such as friends and relatives or direct application off the street, are used at somewhat lower rates yet yield over half of the jobs. A person who relies on ineffective methods risks exhausting energy and patience before getting an offer. Indeed, the success rates for some of the formal methods listed is so low (8% or less of users find a job through the method) that it is questionable whether resorting to them can properly be termed job-seeking.

Setting a timetable completes inital planning and, as with sound advice on sources of leads, can avoid pitfalls. The person must be willing to persist long enough to find a good job and not merely take the first offer that comes along or settle for no job at all. Job search for most people is long on disappointments and short on rewards. The incentives to continue looking despite frustration must come from the counselor or other persons in the job-seeker's life. The job-seeker should recognize that persistence itself speaks well of personal character and worth. For too many clients job search consists of checking one or two leads provided by the counselor, registering with the employment service, reading the want ads, and giving up after 2 weeks, convinced they are failures. Job search often extends 1½ months or more for qualified persons without disabilities (Rosenfeld, 1975). A timetable framed accordingly can prepare the person for the activity involved, shape realistic expectations, and establish a sustainable pace.

COUNSELOR RESPONSIBILITY

Taking a deliberate approach to placement does not mean that the counselor does all of the work. Many, if not most, persons can be prepared to find jobs on their own, and doing so increases the chances that they might move to better jobs or find a new job should the first one be lost. Studies indicate that about half of the persons served by state agencies locate jobs on their own (Samuelson and McPhee, 1963; Mangum and Glenn, 1967; Zadny and James, 1977) and large caseloads in state agencies can preclude intensive counselor involvement. Indeed, the concepts of rehabilitation and of returning persons to the vocational mainstream entail persons with disabilities achieving the same degree of independence in bidding for jobs as persons without disabilities. There are few reasons to suppose that a well-prepared person with a disability will be any less persuasive than the counselor, especially in view of the fact that counselor intervention inherently raises the question of why the job-seeker could not personally handle applying. As Salomone (1971; Salomone and Usdane, 1977) points out, being responsible for placement does not require being a rehabilitation salesperson, but it does involve charting the course of job search, seeing that a person is equipped to look for work, and monitoring progress. Planning is part of fulfilling that responsibility.

Many counselors dislike placement because they consider it unprofessional (Hagan, Haug, and Sussman, 1975). The perception is accurate if the task is handled haphazardly. Professionalism denotes the possession of a specialized body of knowledge and its skillful application to resolve practical problems. Understanding of placement has progressed far enough to meet the first requirement. Planning of services can see that the second is met.

PLANNING FOR PLACEMENT: AN ILLUSTRATION

Deliberately planning for placement is certainly not a new concept. Counselors, as individuals, have implemented their own planning techniques for years. However, there has been little attention given to systematically implementing placement planning practices and studying their impact on placements over an agency or program-wide basis. Only a few agencies and programs have tried to use a system that incorporates formalized placement planning. Since little has been found in the literature to guide individuals in devising the elements important for planning for placement, there is confusion regarding not only whether to plan, but also what should be planned for.

Table 3 illustrates a planning form that has been developed for use in agencies and programs that require separate placement plans. Further research needs to uncover what elements are important when considering placement plans. However, until such information is available, this plan is an example that others may use to guide their own planning efforts. The plan of Table 3 illustrates how a financial needs assessment can guide job lead selection as well as provide an indication of the suitability of a person's potential for acquiring a job that will be financially satisfactory. The congruence between financial needs and earning capability may be useful for predicting a person's motivation for the job search. The plan also provides a graphic illustration that a job search can be expected to last for at least 6 weeks. This can help job searchers to have realistic expectations of the time and effort needed to conduct an efficient job search.

Placement planning should also highlight the important cost factor associated with the job search. There are many potential hidden costs that may lessen a person's initial job search enthusiasm. Transportation costs, child-care needs, foregone leisure time, and clothing costs, among others, have to be expected and handled if the job search is to be practical. Possibly, a counselor can find additional resources to carry job searchers over these cost barriers.

Additionally, systematic planning for placement should lead to a more direct job search: one that minimizes inefficiency and drain on the job searcher's energy. Appropriate labor markets should be carefully identified in advance. Counselors can use the planning routine to teach job-search preparation skills to their clients, thus enabling them to pursue future job search when unemployment occurs or when advancement is desired. Finally, careful planning will help counselors more easily manage large caseloads so their personal energies can be directed toward those clients who will have greater difficulties dealing with the labor market.

Table 3.   Client placement plan

Client name_____ Counselor #_____ Date_____

Client #_____

Instructions: Counselor and client to complete this plan after the client reaches Status 12, but before Status 20. Distribution: One copy to case record and one copy to Central Office. Please review the IWRP at this time.

Total dollar amount of current benefits	$__ __ __
D.O.T. of occupation for which client is being prepared (four digits)	__ __ __ __
Expected salary of this position (weekly)	$__ __ __ __
D.O.T. of alternative occupation (four digits)	__ __ __ __
Expected salary of alternative occupation (weekly)	$__ __ __ __

Steps taken to teach job seeking skills:

_____

_____

Plans to improve specific problems such as transportation, child care, or job engineering:

_____

List possible employers, starting with those who are most likely to have openings for the client.

Name	Address	Phone
_____	_____	_____
_____	_____	_____
_____	_____	_____
_____	_____	_____
_____	_____	_____

Sources of leads to be checked by client:

( ) Family and friends   ( ) Yellow pages
( ) Unions   ( ) Want ads
( ) Former employers   ( ) Employment service
( ) School or training facility ( ) Private employment agency
    placement office   ( ) Other: Specify_____
( ) Going directly to companies
    whether or not they are   _____
    advertising openings
( ) CETA

Table 3. (*Continued*)

Job search plan (6 weeks)

Week 1:   Counselor _____

 Client _____

Week 2:   Counselor _____

 Client _____

Week 3:   Counselor _____

 Client _____

Week 4:   Counselor _____

 Client _____

Week 5:   Counselor _____

 Client _____

Week 6:   Counselor _____

 Client _____

| _____ | _____ | By initialing this, the client agrees that he |
| Counselor initial | Client initial | helped develop this plan and will do his part toward carrying it out. He further understands it is a plan of services that is not legally binding. |

These suggestions for plans are offered only as examples. Counselors, because of their experience, specialized caseloads, and unique settings may find them to be somewhat inappropriate. Until more evidence is at hand to guide the formation of plans, counselors and agencies should be flexible as they gain expertise in placement plan development.

REFERENCES

Hagan, F. E., Haug, M. R., and Sussman, M. B. 1975. Comparative profiles of the rehabilitation counseling graduate: 1965 and 1972. Working Paper No. 5, 2nd Series. Case Western Reserve University, Cleveland, Ohio.

Hamilton, G. S., and Roessner, J. D. 1972. How employers screen disadvantaged job applicants. Monthly Labor Rev. 95(9):14–21.

Jaffe, A. J., Day, L. H., and Adams, W. 1964. Disabled Workers in the Labor Market. Bedminster Press, Totowas, New Jersey.

Keith, R. D., Engelkes, J. R., and Winborn, B. B. 1977. Employment-seeking preparation and activity: An experimental job-placement training model for rehabilitation clients. Rehab. Counsel. Bull. 21(2):159–165.

McClure, D. 1972. Placement through improvement of client's job-seeking skills. J. Appl. Rehab. Counsel. 3(3):188–190.

Mangum, G., and Glenn, L. 1967. Vocational Rehabilitation and Federal Manpower Policy. Institute for Labor and Industrial Relations, Ann Arbor, Michigan.

Ninth Institute of Rehabilitation Services. 1971. Placement and follow-up in the vocational rehabilitation process. DHEW Social and Rehabilitation Services. San Antonio. DHEW Pub. No. (SRS) 72-25007.

Rosenfeld, C. 1975. Job-seeking methods used by American workers. Monthly Labor Rev. August:39–42.

Salomone, P. R. 1971. A client-centered approach to job placement. Voc. Guid. Quart. 19:266–270.

Salomone, P. R., and Usdane, W. M. 1977. Client-centered placement revisited: A dialogue on placement philosophy. Rehab. Counsel. Bull. 21(2):85–91.

Samuelson, C. O., and McPhee, W. 1963. The utility of the rehabilitation process. Rehab. Counsel. Bull. 7:49–53.

Thoreson, R. W., Smits, S. J., Butler, A. J., and Wright, G. H. 1968. Counselor problems associated with client characteristics. Wisconsin Studies in Vocational Rehabilitation, Monograph III. University of Wisconsin Regional Rehabilitation Research Institute, Madison, Wisconsin.

Veglahn, P. A. 1975. Job search patterns of paraplegics. Rehab. Counsel. Bull. 20:129–136.

Zadny, J. J., and James, L. F. 1977. Job placement of the vocationally handicapped: A survey of technique. Studies in Placement, Monograph No. 2. Regional Rehabilitation Research Institute, Portland State University, Portland, Oregon.

Zadny, J. J., and James, L. F. 1978. A survey of job search patterns among state vocational rehabilitation clients. Rehab. Counsel. Bull. 22:60–65.

Zadny, J. J., and James, L. F. The problem with placement. Rehab. Counsel. Bull. In press.

Chapter 5

Placement as Brokerage

*Information Problems
in the Labor Market
for Rehabilitated Workers*

Mark Granovetter

Editor's note: This chapter shows how a counselor can be a broker of labor market information. The counselor has played this role in the development of the Individualized Written Rehabilitation Plan. Intimate knowledge of both the service user and service providers in the community enables the counselor to inform the client of the availability of certain services. At the same time, the counselor can give information about the client to potential service providers so that providers can determine suitability for services.

Professor Granovetter suggests that this brokerage function should be expanded at the placement stage. Counselors are in the best position to give employers accurate information about client's work readiness and qualifications for a job. Counselors who work with employers are also in an excellent position to keep clients abreast of local labor market conditions.

There is much practical advice given. For example, the information a counselor gives to an employer may not be totally unbiased, but if a counselor wishes to do repeat "business" with an employer, it is in the counselor's interest to provide accurate information.

The author also points out the most effective sources of job information and presents empirical evidence to back his claim that the shorter an information chain, the more productive it will be. He presents a rationale for employer screening behavior.

Professor Granovetter says more attention must be paid to the economics and sociology of vocational rehabilitation. His research also challenges neo-classical labor theory to some extent in that he implicitly argues that for some job-seekers, labor market information can be costless.

Well-trained vocational rehabilitation counselors are usually exposed to an academic curriculum that puts its main stress on counseling and clinical psychology, motivation, and the particular physical and psychological problems likely to be faced by those who have been in some way "disabled."

Since the end result of rehabilitation programs is meant to be placement of the rehabilitated person, an outsider might imagine that the curriculum would give equal time to understanding the labor market problems to be faced in this task. In fact, labor market problems typically receive little systematic attention. To some extent this is because the problems of information and placement in the labor market have only in recent years become the subject of theoretical academic speculation. The purpose of this chapter is to review and summarize these recent developments in economics and sociology and discuss their implications for the theory and practice of vocational rehabilitation.

THE IDEA OF A "LABOR MARKET"

Economists have long assumed that, in principle, labor could be analyzed in the same way as other commodities. In the "perfect market" of classical and neoclassical economics there are producers and consumers. Farmers know how much wheat, for example, to produce at any prevailing price. Naturally, the higher the price, the more they produce. Consumers know how much wheat to purchase at any given price; the higher the price, the less they consume. When there is complete information, i.e., everyone knows who is producing and consuming how much, the interplay of these "supply" and "demand" forces guarantees that the same amount is produced as consumed. This market is said to be in "equilibrium."

This account summarizes the "wheat market." In the "labor market," "labor" is the "commodity" to be bought and sold. The price of labor is wages. Workers are the "producers" of labor, and will offer more labor at higher wages than at lower ones; employers are the "consumers" of labor, and will demand more as the wage that needs to be paid is lower. In the market for wheat or for labor, it is assumed that no single producer or consumer has a large enough segment of the market to have any material impact on the price. Thus, both the farmer who produces wheat and the consumer who buys it are simply faced with a price that has been set as a result of market forces beyond their control. All they can adjust is how much they produce or consume. Similarly, at least in the idealized case, neither employer nor employee has much control over what the "going wage" is for a particular type or quality of labor. The employer can adjust how many workers are hired and the worker how many hours are to be given to work.

The reader not previously exposed to the theory of labor markets must by now have imagined a series of objections to this account. Most of these objections concern *information difficulties*. Producers and consumers of wheat may well be aware of each other and of how much wheat is being produced and consumed. In the "labor market," however, we know that it is often hard to ferret out who is hiring and who is available to be hired. Furthermore, the seller of wheat does not much care to whom the sale is made; the seller of labor is entering into an ongoing association with the employer, and cares a great deal about whether this employer and job are suitable.

On the buyer's side, the quality of wheat is easy to determine; but employers, the purchasers of labor, find it hard to judge the quality of labor offered by a particular individual. The standard theory of wages assumes that employers are profit-maximizers, and therefore set an individual's wages according to "productivity"—the extent to which the employee enhances the firm's production (see, for example, Rees, 1973). Until recently, little theoretical attention was given to how employers could or did figure out how productive a given worker *was*.

The prevailing attitude among economists about information problems in labor markets, until around 1960, was that they were unfortunate "imperfections" in the market process and that they impeded the efficient allocation of labor. The problem to be solved was how such imperfections could be gotten rid of; the possibility that they might be inescapable, given the type of market, was not taken seriously. For example, a long series of local labor market studies carried out from the 1930s on showed that formal means of job placement, such as employment agencies and services and newspapers advertisements, generally accounted for only a small proportion of actual hires—rarely more than 20%. Rather, the bulk of the placements were accounted for by information gotten by friends and relatives and "blind" or "gate" applications. The labor economists who discovered this generally considered it an example of irrational behavior, which could be made to go away by proper applications of public policy.

In the early 1960s, the tide in economics began to turn. Two articles by the Chicago economist George Stigler (1961, 1962) were particularly influential. The most crucial point made in these articles was that *information is not free*. In order to get information, people need to expend time, effort, and, frequently, money. Information, therefore, has many of the characteristics of other scarce commodities and can thus be made a proper subject of economic analysis. If producers or consumers require information, Stigler argued, they will obtain it as they would any other commodity, paying the required price (i.e., incurring the required costs) only up to the point where the benefits expected from the information still exceed the costs. In the case of labor markets, Stigler focused on the costs of "job search" to workers. A further dimension was added to this discussion by the economist Albert Rees, who made the distinction between "extensive" and "intensive" searches. In a market where the product is highly standardized, one needs mainly to search extensively—to find out who *all* the buyers or sellers are. If, however, the quality of the product is highly variable, an intensive search is more appropriate. The need in this case is not so much to find all the buyers or sellers, but rather to find some who look promising and then find out more about what each one has to offer. The market for new cars, for example, is one in which consumers are well advised to make an extensive search. In the market for *used* cars, however, appearance is generally not to be trusted, and the buyer wants to know as much as he can about a few good possibilities to avoid being stuck with a "lemon." The relevant point here is that the labor market is precisely the kind of market that requires intensive searches for information; prospective jobs as well as prospective employees may appear promising but can turn out to be "lemons" (see Rees and Shultz, 1970, pp. 200-203).

In the 1970s, the discussion of "job search" was complemented by a consideration of how employers read the applicants' "signals," which might indicate how productive they would be on the job. As in the literature on how workers get information about jobs, economists emphasized that there is a cost to be borne if the employer is to get good information about how productive a given employee is—this is the other side of the "intensive" search process. The cost may be borne by the employer, who might use elaborate testing and screening devices. It may also be incurred by the prospective employee, who invests money and time in certification devices that supposedly inform the employer of productivity. Economists have proposed that getting educational degrees is an investment of this kind for employees (see Spence, 1974).

A sociological dimension was added to this discussion by a study of a random sample of job-changers in a Boston suburb (Granovetter, 1974). It is neither accidental nor irrational that both workers and employers actually *prefer* to get information about prospective jobs or employees through personal contacts rather than by way of more formal procedures—a result found not only in this study, but also by decades of labor economists. This preference can best be understood in the context of the costs and benefits of information: a) information gotten through personal contacts is less costly to obtain than by other means, in terms of both time and effort, and b) such information is also of better *quality* than that received from formal sources: "a friend gives more than a simple job-description—he may also indicate if prospective workmates are congenial, if the boss is neurotic, and if the company is moving forward or is stagnant . . . Similarly . . . evaluations of prospective employees will be trusted better when the employer knows the evaluator personally" (Granovetter, 1974, p. 13).

Information from advertisements, agencies, or résumés, by contrast, is harder to trust. The searcher or employer will naturally assume that these sources are trying to put the best face on the situation and have no strong motive for complete honesty. One standard way employers have of getting information they trust is to recruit through current employees. Labor economists Rees and Shultz (1970) comment that the "strong employer preference for employee referrals requires some explanation in view of the general hostility of labor economists to unorganized markets and to informal channels of transmitting market information. . . . The greater the variance in the quality or nature of the item or service to be traded, the greater are the inherent obstacles to the formal organization of markets, and the larger the amount of intensive search that may be needed. . . . Employee referrals are very well suited to providing qualitative information to both parties. An employer who is satisfied with his work force is likely to get new employees similar to those he already has. He may feel that the reputation of his present employees is to some extent at stake when they make referrals, and that they will therefore have an incentive to recommend people who in their judgment would do well" (pp. 201, 203).

INFORMATION PROBLEMS IN THE
LABOR MARKET FOR REHABILITATED WORKERS

The preceding theoretical material leads up to the main argument: information problems in the labor market for rehabilitated workers are even more complex than in ordinary labor markets. These problems require special and explicit treatment in terms of needs and expectations of both client or job-seeker and employer.

The employer's information problem is to figure out how "productive" an employee would be if hired—that is, what would the applicant add to the firm's output. (A useful view of the entire rehabilitation process as one of "productivity enrichment" is provided in Vandergoot, Jacobsen, and Worrall, this volume). Employers generally believe that "on paper," almost anyone can be made to appear productive. When faced with many thousands of applications for a position, then, the sorting problem becomes almost hopeless, and the process becomes potentially prohibitive in cost. Reliance by employers on their personal contacts is one way out of this dilemma; this system cuts down the number of prospects and improves the information about each. Another widely used expedient is the elimination of large categories of individuals from the process; a typical example is the insistence that applicants be high school graduates. It has been strongly argued that such a requirement is frequently only vaguely related to actual job performance. Berg (1970) describes the notion that education increases productivity as the "great training robbery." Dore (1976) is even more graphic, entitling his book *The Diploma Disease*.

This strategy of eliminating potential applicants can be viewed as designating people without the proper educational credentials as ipso facto "handicapped." It is thus not surprising that many employers might add to their screening strategy the requirement that applicants have no *physical* impairment. The analogy shows that in discriminating against those with physical disabilities, employers may not be implementing some deep-seated emotional prejudice against people, say, in wheelchairs, or with physical impairments, but merely adopting another screening device that will lower their information costs. The distinction is an important one for policy purposes. If the discrimination resulted from a deep-seated prejudice, the best policy prescription would be a massive educational campaign to inform employers that people with disabilities are "normal" in most respects, so that hiring them is "good business." If it results from a general screening strategy, then such a broad campaign would be no more effective than trying to convince employers that hiring the undereducated was "good business." What would likely work instead would be to convey to particular employers high-quality information about the suitability of *particular* workers with disabilities, for particular jobs or types of jobs.

The more specific information available about individuals, the less likely would an employer view them as a member of some preconceived category. Thus, Hart (1962) comments that it is "not uncommon for an employer to state with sincerity that he does not have any handicapped employees, and to reveal later . . . that he does have a man with one eye, another with a leg brace, and another who is illiterate. . . . One placement supervisor . . . asked a plant superintendent if he ever hired any retardates. The reaction was a glare and: 'This is a nice shop. We don't employ people like that here.' Actually, he did have retardates working there, but he never thought of them in these terms" (p. 35).

If "education" is required for employers at all, it should take the form of explaining that certain types of disabilities actually lead to *higher*, not lower, productivity in some jobs. Persons who are severely retarded, traditionally difficult to place, may well be a boon to employers in jobs that normally have high turnover. MacDonald (1974) suggests asking employers which jobs have such turnover, since "many jobs hav-

ing a high turnover rate make ideal initial placement opportunities for
our clients . . . Many . . . are hard to keep filled because as soon as possible the person who stays on finds a way to another department or gains
additional skills and begins to move up the ladder" (pp. 6-7). Hart
(1962) suggests a comment on the order of "'That seems to be a very
monotonous job. I don't suppose a bright person would last doing that
day after day?' We have been able in this way to ease into a discussion of
people who have not gone very far in school and cannot read or write,
but can do physical labor or repetitive work and are more likely to stick
to such jobs than better educated people" (p. 35).

Because employers typically prefer to hire individuals about whom
they have information from personal sources, the possibility cannot be
ruled out that there is actually no discrimination against people with
disabilities because of their disabilities. Rather, the discrimination may
result when these workers are presented to employers impersonally,
through agencies. It is well documented that employers distrust agencies
of all kinds. The rehabilitation agency has an advantage, in principle: far
richer information about a client may be made available to employers
than could be given by a state or private employment service about one
of its clients. Contact is much more intimate and prolonged between
client and agency when rehabilitation has taken place than in any other
situation. To the extent, however, that the placement function is shunted
to the "end of the service delivery line" (Usdane, 1976, p. 163), resulting
information about clients given to employers may look pretty much
the same.

To know the actual level of discrimination against the disabled
would require information on the relative success of those disabled who
hunt jobs on their own, especially through personal contacts, compared
to those who hunt mainly through agencies. Such data are not easily
available, since most of what we know about the disabled is the result of
their contact with agencies. Some of what might be found is suggested by
a study carried out by Jaffee, Day, and Adams (1964) of a cross section
of workers with serious and permanent disabilities as a result of job-
related injuries in the New York metropolitan area. Fully two-thirds of
the workers studied subsequently returned to work with the previous
employers. Such a return is an interesting special case of what happens
when an employer has good quality information about a worker with a
disability. In this case, the information is viewed by the employer as the
best available since it does not rely at all on intermediaries, but is rather
the result of a particular worker having been actually observed on the job
and personally known before the disability. It is possible to speculate that
the same worker, with the disability, would have a much harder time trying to find a *new* employer for whom the most salient characteristic

might become the disability rather than any actual capability to produce. Nagi, McBroom, and Collette (1972) comment that "even ex-mental patients, who seem to have relatively low employment rates, are reported to have been often rehired by former employers . . . knowledge about the impaired person, his skills and work habits reduces the situational ambiguity and limits stereotypical responses" (p. 23). The workers with disabilities themselves, of course, also have difficult information problems in the labor market. Most of the usual disabilities increase the cost to the worker of gathering information about job openings. If the disability is of comparatively recent origin, the worker is apt to be confused about what actual abilities remain compared to what they were. The worker needs guidance about what now would constitute a suitable job. Most people would find it difficult, however, to broach such questions openly to a prospective employer. To do so would constitute admission that the applicant might well not be suitable for whatever openings exist. This problem is particularly acute for the worker who has been disabled in such a way that a previous occupation is no longer a practical alternative.

REHABILITATION AGENCIES AS INFORMATION RESOURCES

It is well known that rehabilitation agencies provide crucial services to their clients. Another way to view such agencies and their personnel should be stressed: as information intermediaries for persons with disabilities in the labor market. If it is true, as argued here, that information costs for employers and job-searchers in the market for workers with disabilities are even higher than in ordinary labor markets, then rehabilitation agencies are in a unique position to reduce those costs on both sides of the market.

One may ask why these agencies should be in the business of reducing employer costs, given that employers are not the "clients" who are to be served. The answer is that employers are economic actors, interested in minimizing their costs and maximizing productivity. To the extent that an agency can help an employer do that, the employer will be strongly motivated to hire its clients; it will be "good business" because employer search costs will be reduced and quality information about the prospective employee will be available.

No one is in a better position to offer reliable information about the strengths and weaknesses of a rehabilitated worker than the organization that has had the main part in planning and carrying out his rehabilitation. This does not by any means guarantee that such information will be accepted as gospel. Employers are distrustful of information from sources with which they are not personally acquainted. They suspect that unless the information comes from a source with whom they have some meaningful continuing relationship, the source has little motive to be entirely honest. Moreover, without knowledge of the informant, the employer has no way of knowing how good an agency is at understanding particular work requirements or at screening individuals. Employers do not generally get good information from either private or public employment agencies because the clients and "counselors" of those agencies have only a transient relationship. Hence, the agency's knowledge of each client is extremely limited; moreover, in most such organizations employees are paid or promoted according to the number of placements. Thus, there is neither the ability nor the motive to offer high-quality information. The situation is quite different in most rehabilitation agencies, but employers who have not had direct experience with a given agency have no way of knowing this.

Just as rehabilitation agencies are uniquely positioned to reduce information costs to employers, they are also in the best position to do so for their clients. In principle, at least, the agency has the resources to do what would be prohibitively expensive and difficult for its clients to do. It can make a thorough survey of the local labor market to acquire a detailed understanding of exactly what kinds of jobs are tenable for those with various kinds of disabilities and find out where job openings are likely to occur. Through continuing contact with specific employers the agency is in a position to provide information about particular openings appropriate for particular clients.

PROBLEMS OF IMPLEMENTATION

To say that rehabilitation agencies are in a unique *position* to serve as intermediaries capable of reducing information costs in the labor market for people with disabilities is not to imply that this happens automatically. To accomplish this it is necessary for individuals who have detailed knowledge about a particular worker to *convey* this knowledge to employers, and for someone who has detailed knowledge of both the worker and the labor market to assist the worker in finding suitable work. In practice, there seems to be a good deal of resistance to serving these functions on the part of rehabilitation counselors, who are logically in the best position to do so. Hart and Karbott (1964) remark, for example, on the "attitude of so many (counselors) upon their arrival from the university to their place of employment. When it is suggested that they visit employers and see jobs, their answers so often mean, though they may use other words: 'I am a counselor and I use my time counseling, and I do not have the time to visit employers. Somebody else should do that'" (p. 10).

To understand the genesis of this attitude, it is useful to review the history of the profession of rehabilitation counseling. Sussman's account (1965, pp. 179–222) is especially illuminating. He pays particular attention to the problems such counselors have had in establishing a professional identity: "Until very recently, rehabilitation was largely unknown . . . Even today, . . . the layman is for the most part unfamiliar with the field, those who work in it, and the tasks they perform. . . . The consequence is extensive variability in the perception of the field and the workers within it. . . . Part of the socialization of childhood is playing occupational games such as 'What would you like to be: nurse, teacher, doctor, lawyer?' . . . How many parents ever ask, 'do you want to be a rehabilitation worker?' or more specifically, a 'vocational rehabilitation counselor?'" (p. 210). Sussman argues further that the word *vocational* suggests "the kind of instruction found in training schools for noncollege bound youth. It has a lower-class connotation." One way to offset this connotation is "to use as little as possible the term 'vocational' in designating the work objectives of the counselor . . . Another tack is to stress the counseling activity of the job" (pp. 210–211).

Sussman also notes that people involved in newly developing occupations try to establish professional identity in a way that will increase their autonomy, status, and rewards. "Professionalism and generally higher-status occupational positions have been associated with 'clean' work. . . . In contrast, 'dirty' work has been allied with low status and nonprofessional jobs. It is the work that someone has to do; the society cannot exist without it, and it may be 'dirty' in either the physical or psychological sense or both" (p. 195). He adds, "Within the counseling role, certain tasks are considered less desirable than others. Finding a job for the handicapped worker is considered the least professional and is most disturbing to the counselor. This may be in part due to the higher number of employer refusals and the attendant frustrations and in part to the counselor's confrontation of the meaning of the handicap and the repugnance to it expressed by society. The counselor . . . closes out the rest of the world as he moves the client along the counseling trail. In time he must emerge and face the reality of the 'dirty work' of his calling" (pp. 216–217).

Even those who believe counselors should take an active part in placement acknowledge that the job is frequently seen as dirty work. This is especially stressed by those who advocate counselor separation from placement (e.g., Salomone, 1971). Salomone gives one reason why counselors should not actively engage in placement work: "they are not trained to be salesmen" (p. 267). This comment relates clearly to Sussman's discussion of professionalism. The implication is that sales is dirty work, of lower status than counseling. It conjures up the image of a vacuum cleaner peddler shoving his foot in the door and throwing dirt on the carpet to facilitate the demonstration of his wares. Selling *is* an occupation of low autonomy: one's personality is on the line all the time, and results depend entirely on others' decisions. Much of one's workday is spent in the nonproductive and uninteresting activity of traveling from one prospective buyer to another. In Arthur Miller's well-known play "Death of a Salesman," the protagonist, Willy Loman, is even given a name—"low man"—that explicitly reflects this social status.

How can this problem be overcome? One approach has been to sidestep the "dirty work" issue and stress the rewarding aspects of placement. Hart and Karbott (1964), for example, argue that each

> visit to a business concern brings a counselor new knowledge and sharpens interest and understanding . . . Nameless buildings which the counselor once heedlessly rushed by on his way to the office or on visits to clinics become places of fascination when he investigates and in various rooms finds small companies polishing industrial diamonds, clipping items for newspapers, assembling telescopes, dunning debtors, making dentures, framing pictures and sewing on lamp shades. Deep satisfaction arises from sharing this knowledge with clients and from making actual placements (p. 10).

These arguments should not be shrugged off; yet they have some of the quality of Tom Sawyer's explanation of why it is fun to whitewash a fence. The idea that placement is low-status, dirty work will not disappear and must be faced head on.

The kind of theoretical framework that has developed in recent years in the sociology and economics of information can make an important contribution to the redefinition of placement and job development. It can do this in part because the prestige of any activity is related, perhaps more than it should be, to the presence or absence of theoretical and academic underpinnings justifying it. This appears to be one reason why the model of the rehabilitation counselor as a species of counseling psychologist achieved such widespread approval following World War II. Counseling psychology was a recognized specialty, and the rehabilitation counselor identified with this specialty could be more readily treated as a professional than someone whose activities were not known to require professional training (see Sussman, 1965, pp. 212–214). Successful placement workers, on the other hand, might be seen as clever, but not professional. Usdane (1976) comments that many such workers have "found that the 'little black book' of names, addresses, firms, contacts, relatives and other social sources successfully placed handicapped people. But . . . advancement within the placement area is minimal. As a result, management, supervision or higher pay in regular counseling positions restrain the person from continuing what has been a creditable performance and service to the handicapped. Another novice then repeats the placement learning process on the job, and the cycle continues" (p. 166). The counselor then is seen as doing something that requires substantial training. The use of a "little black book" hardly seems to merit the same approval; it is too informal, too much like what a salesperson might do. Seeing placement and job development work as a specialty in information services and brokerage, on the other hand, gives an entirely different connotation to the job. The successful placement worker is not just a fast-talking salesperson, but rather a professional, trained in economics and sociology.

Nor is this new conception merely a smoke screen, which redefines the same old activity in a new way. An understanding of these theoretical notions should tell us that the old salesperson image is not really a useful description of placement work. In the economic and sociological ideas reported here, emphasis is placed on the *quality* of information sought by employers and potential employees. This quality can be achieved only through a *continuing* personal relationship between the producer and consumer of information. Hence, the word *broker* conveys a more accurate image than *salesperson*. Rather than suggesting a one-time encounter between buyer and seller, the word *broker* describes an individual who is seen as continuously providing a valuable service to two sides of a transaction—a professional who, whatever type of brokerage is involved, brings together buyers and sellers and absorbs much of the cost they would otherwise have had to incur in finding an appropriate match.

The stress on continuity is important. If an agency is set up in such a way that a particular source of placement information never sees the same employer more than once, the latter will reasonably wonder how strong the motivation can be to give him accurate information about a client to be placed. In a continuing relationship, however, one knows that future placements will be jeopardized by giving poor information for the sake of a current one. In the end, all parties gain from the ensuing development of trust.

Good brokerage requires intimate knowledge of *both* sides of the market in which the broker acts as liaison. This means not only knowing the client and his needs well, but also having detailed understanding of the workplaces where placement attempts are made. Since the information an employer needs concerns how productive a particular client would be in his workplace, it is clear that the placement worker will be unable to say anything intelligent about this in the absence of a thorough understanding of exactly what kind of work goes on in that setting. Since many jobs do not result from "vacancies" but rather from an opening being created for the "right" person, an important part of the brokerage can involve seeing that a certain client has exactly the right skills that an employer needs. Without close knowledge of all sides of the market, such creative brokerage cannot take place. Job development, as well as placement, then falls under the same analysis.

PLACEMENT BY WHOM?

Professionalism is not the only issue involved in arguments that placement is not the counselor's job. Counselors, it may be asserted, have neither the time nor the proper training for placement work. The specialty of placement can be seen as sufficiently distinct from counseling that it ought to involve specific training for special personnel in rehabilitation agencies. Usdane (1976) argues, for example, that to "reinforce the importance of this particular area of important service, there needs to be developed professionally a new professional, the Placement Worker. Training should be at the graduate level in a department of either economics or business administration" (p. 166). In a number of states, placement specialists have worked at a "district" level, which is more centralized than that of the local VR agency, engaging in job development projects and giving technical placement assistance to counselors. Although such specialists place workers themselves, their main function seems to be coordinating placement activities and educating counselors in the problems of job placement. (For details see Lillehaugen, 1964, on Minnesota; Molinaro, 1977, on Michigan; Hart and Karbott, 1964, on Massachusetts). Thus, the idea of a "team" effort is often suggested. The placement specialist makes sure that part of the rehabilitation process itself is finding a job for the person with a disability.

It may well be that such a division of labor, with different specialists overseeing different aspects of rehabilitation, can be more efficient than trying to make the counselor a jack-of-all trades. Whether such a division of labor is needed probably depends on caseloads and the particular kind of disabilities and labor markets faced by any particular rehabilitation facility or agency. Although generalization is difficult, one may safely say that there is a danger in giving all the responsibility for placement to specialists. Such specialists could become too distant from clients, and the quality of information they are able to offer about them to employers would naturally suffer. For employers, the most believable and reliable information about potential employees will come from those individuals who know the applicants best, that is, those who have planned and implemented their rehabilitation programs. If a system becomes so bureaucratized that job descriptions move along through a highly centralized facility, past several intermediaries to the local counselor and then names move back up this chain, credibility is liable to vanish. In a study of how a general random sample of professional technical and managerial workers found jobs (Granovetter, 1974, pp. 51–62), the length of the chains of contact between the initial source of the information (the employer) and the person who subsequently took the job was of some importance. If, for example, A heard about a job from B, who heard about it from C, who heard about it from D, who heard about it from E, who heard about it from the employer, then there are four information intermediaries in this information chain. In fact, the study found that chains of length four accounted for *none* of the job information found by the respondents, and that over 96% reported that the information chain that led to their jobs (among those whose jobs were found through personal contacts—the majority of respondents) was of length two or less. Of these, most chains were of length either zero (i.e., no intermediaries; respondent heard directly from the employer) or one. Only one of eight had a chain of length two.

The reason for this seems to lie in the different quality of information received by employers through chains of different lengths. The best information is obtained when the employer actually knows the prospective employee (chain length zero). Excellent information may also be obtained by the employer through some trusted intermediary who knows the prospective employee well (chain length one). When there are two intermediaries, there is already someone in the information chain with whom the employer is not personally acquainted: he thus has difficulty deciding whether to trust the information. The unknown person in this case is crucial, too, since that individual is the one who knows the prospective employee. Beyond lengths of two, employers have no reason to value the information received any more highly than if it came through entirely impersonal sources. "Just as reading about a job in the newspaper affords me no recommendation in applying for it, neither does it to have heard about it fifth-hand" (Granovetter, 1974, p. 59).

The significance of these considerations in organizing the placement role is clear; insofar as placement specialists are used at all, they will be valuable to the degree that they are in personal touch with the individuals they will place. This argues strongly for a conception of such a specialist not as someone who comes in at the end of rehabilitation as part of a "mop-up" operation, but rather as someone whose skills are made an integral part of the rehabilitation process from beginning to end.

CLIENT-CENTERED PLACEMENT AND CLIENT SELF-ESTEEM

It is not only argued that counselors should not be involved in placement because it is "unprofessional" and because counselors do not have the time, but also because counselor involvement in placement discourages self-reliance on the part of the client. Salomone (1971), for example, arguing for "client-centered placement," believes that "the counselor

who secures a definite job lead for his client may place his client successfully but in the process may limit client satisfaction and pride associated
with locating and obtaining one's own job . . . Clients who have not
engaged in their own successful job-hunting practices are likely to return,
again and again, to the counselor for additional selective placement
services." In "client-centered placement," by contrast, the client is
required "to assume the major responsibility for securing job leads, for
contacting employers, and for performing the necessary follow-up
activities . . ." (1971, p. 267). The counselor's role is that of teaching the
client "all the major factors related to successful job seeking" (1971,
p. 268).

If one takes the economic and sociological arguments raised in this
chapter seriously, such an assertion is difficult to accept. Salamone,
consistent with the clinical psychology orientation and training characteristic of the counseling profession, implicitly assumes that the main
problems for the client are motivational and personal. Such an approach
implies that once a client is self-reliant and has learned the right job-
hunting "procedures," he will be readily employable. In the ordinary
labor market, things do not work out that way. For workers without
disabilities, the better jobs go to those who find jobs through personal
contacts (Granovetter, 1974, pp. 13–14). Even those who do not have an
impairment to explain away do relatively worse in the job search if their
job information comes through impersonal sources; it helps if someone
"fills in" the employer about them in a reliable way. The vocationally
rehabilitated worker who has no such personal route to the employer
ends up even further behind the eight ball than a worker without an
impairment. If rehabilitation has involved extensive retraining, then it is
highly unlikely that the worker will have useful personal contacts left
over from previous work experience. Those contacts would know mainly
about work of a different kind from that which is now feasible. Under
such circumstances, it seems particularly unwise for the only people who
have reliable information for employers—the counselor and others who
were involved in rehabilitation—to adopt a "hands off" attitude in order
to build self-reliance. Such a proposal reflects a failure to understand
problems of information and recruitment in functioning labor markets.
In most cases, it would only put clients at a disadvantage compared to
those without disabilities who find good jobs not because they are so
"skilled" at job-seeking, but because they have appropriate contacts.

This is not to say that counselors should not assist clients in preparing for interviews by using such techniques as role-playing, or by suggesting "appropriate appearance and mannerisms" (Salomone, 1971, p. 268).
Other techniques of building self-reliance certainly can be encouraged as
well, such as the "job-finding clubs" developed by Jones and Azrin

(1973). The argument here is simply that such procedures will generally be insufficient compensation for the disadvantage most rehabilitated workers face in their initial entry to the labor market. Some attempt must be made to convey reasonably accurate information to employers about specific individuals. Such information will not be accepted as such in the absence of a continuing personal relationship between rehabilitation agencies and relevant local employers.

Previously placed rehabilitated workers can be valuable potential resources for developing good information about job openings and actual working conditions in a place of employment. It is well understood (if rarely implemented) that those workers who are placed successfully should be followed up carefully to assure that they make a good adjustment to the new work setting, and to determine whether they require additional services. Another, usually unforeseen, advantage of good follow-up is that the successfully placed worker is an extraordinarily valuable potential resource person. The worker is aware of ongoing trends in the work setting, which can be used in adjusting training programs as well as in keeping track of openings. This aspect of follow-up is particularly well suited to building the self-reliance of the former client, because the client becomes a consultant contributing a valuable service, rather than merely seeing himself as someone who may still require assistance. In any given community, a "council" of successfully placed clients may be an unexpectedly useful addition to placement activities of an agency. Such a council could also function to illustrate to those not yet placed that others have "made it" and are now respected citizens in their own right.

SUMMARY

The main point of this chapter has been to argue that in the practice of vocational rehabilitation, too much attention has been paid to psychological and motivational problems and not enough to the economic and sociological theory of those labor markets in which clients must ultimately be placed. This has resulted in part from the dominance of the clinical orientation in the training of counselors, partly from the historical evolution of the counseling profession, and partly from the lack of a well-defined theory of placement problems in economics and sociology. Over the last 10 to 20 years, some of the most interesting developments in labor economics and economic sociology have occurred in the area of information transactions and costs. The advent of this new theoretical apparatus, sketched only briefly here, raises the possibility of a new type of training for those who enter the profession of vocational rehabilitation. Ultimately, the study of such subjects ought to be an important part of standard training in this field. Even before the next generation of vocational rehabilitation workers is trained, these developments can be taken into account in current placement programs. An understanding of how information functions in the usual labor market placement process should help rehabilitation agencies to see more clearly that they are in a position to offer their clients an advantage usually available only to those with contacts in the ordinary labor market: the rehabilitation facility can present a worker to an employer in a way that will be found convincing and trustworthy. This does not put the employer's welfare ahead of the client's; it only acknowledges that the welfare of both parties cannot be artificially separated.

The lack of systematic attention to placement at present decreases the value of the entire rehabilitation experience for clients. It also brings vocational rehabilitation into a weak position in competing for increasingly scarce public funds. In a recent analysis of the economics of rehabilitation programs, Levitan and Taggart (1977) comment: "vocational rehabilitation efforts have been immune from the critical scrutiny leveled at other human resource investments, but a day of reckoning may be at hand. The burden of proof for social welfare spending has increased" (p. xii). They go on to argue that the studies purporting to show unusually high benefit/cost ratios for such programs have relied on faulty methodology, especially in the lack of proper control groups (pp. 75–84).

In the future, then, it will become increasingly necessary for the practitioners of vocational rehabilitation to develop some sophistication about the economic and sociological context in which their work takes place. Better understanding of placement depends on this sophistication. Until this understanding is achieved, employers and an increasingly cost-conscious public will not easily be convinced that rehabilitating people with disabilities is "good business."

REFERENCES

Berg, I. 1970. Education and Jobs: The Great Training Robbery. Beacon Press, Boston.
Dore, R. P. 1976. The Diploma Disease. University of California Press, Berkeley.
Granovetter, M. 1974. Getting a Job: A Study of Contacts and Careers. Harvard University Press, Cambridge, Massachusetts.
Hart, W. 1962. Effective approaches to employers. Rehab. Rec. 3:34–37.
Hart, W. and Karbott, M. 1964. Placement in counselor's job. Rehab. Rec. 5 (1):1–10.
Jaffee, A. J., Day, L., and Adams, W. 1964. Disabled Workers in the Labor Market. Bedminster Press, Totowa, New Jersey.
Jones, P. J., and Azrin, N. 1973. An experimental application of a social rein-

forcement approach to the problem of job-finding. J. Appl. Behav. Anal. 6 (3):345–353.

Levitan, S. A., and Taggart, R. 1977. Jobs for the Disabled. Johns Hopkins Press, Baltimore.

Lillehaugen, S. T. 1964. District placement counselors can boost jobs for handicapped. Rehab. Rec. 5 (2):29–31.

MacDonald, D. J. 1974. The rehabilitation counselor: A resource person to industry; a revitalized approach to selective placement. J. Appl. Rehab. Counsel. 5(1):3–7.

Molinaro, D. 1977. A placement system develops and settles: The Michigan Model. Mimeograph. Human Resources Center, Albertson, N.Y.

Nagi, S. Z., McBroom, W., and Collette, J. 1972. Work, employment and the disabled. Am. J. Econ. Sociol. 31 (1):21–33.

Rees, A. 1973. The Economics of Work and Pay. Harper & Row Publishers, New York.

Rees, A., and Shultz, G. 1970. Workers and Wages in an Urban Labor Market. The University of Chicago Press, Chicago.

Salamone, P. 1971. A client-centered approach to job placement. Voc. Guid. Quart. 19 (4):266–270.

Spence, A. M. 1974. Market Signaling: Information Transfer in Hiring and Related Screening Processes. Harvard University Press, Cambridge, Massachusetts.

Stigler, G. 1961. The economics of information. J. Pol. Econ. 69:213–225.

Stigler, G. 1962. Information in the labor market. J. Pol. Econ. 70 (2): 94–105.

Sussman, M. 1965. Occupational sociology and rehabilitation. In M. Sussman (ed.), Sociology and Rehabilitation, pp. 179–222. American Sociological Association, Washington, D.C.

Usdane, W. M. 1976. The placement process in the rehabilitation of the severely handicapped. Rehab. Lit. 37 (6):162–167.

Chapter 6

Empirically Based Technologies for Job Development

Jesse E. Gordon

Editor's note: Professor Gordon suggests that job developers are responsible for analyzing tasks and identifying new technologies in the jobs they develop. He maintains that such analysis should begin with an examination of the job development function itself. He presents two strategies for introducing empirically based technologies that would take job development beyond the current state of the art. His call for analysis of the job development role and then empirical testing is reminiscent of Dr. Bruyère's contention in Chapter 11 that before training and staff development take place, activities that lead to successful placement must be identified.

The chapter provides a list of tasks that highly productive school placement personnel are likely to perform. The list is suggestive and can be of value to job developers in rehabilitation programs. Professor Gordon also suggests ways in which the introduction of innovations can be enhanced. Counselors, placement specialists, and job developers will find Gordon's generalizations useful in dealing with employers.

Working with employers to develop jobs will enable job developers to expand their information networks. This expansion will lower the costs of job search for prospective rehabilitants and save rehabilitation resources. The employer contacts will also help to provide job developers with ammunition in the battle to get employers to adopt innovations such as, in this case, hiring people with disabilities.

Gordon presents job developers with several challenges: Developers, practice what you preach! Developers, reach out to the social sciences; use what they have to teach, and ground your own field in empiricism.

Do not envy job developers in rehabilitation. Consider:

1. Trained in motivational/emotional counseling of persons with disabilities, they perform tasks that have low status and prestige. Job developers are not even considered professional by others involved in rehabilitation work.

2. Adding injury to insult, job developers' tasks tend to be judged by a fairly simple counting of outcomes. Because of this, any evaluation of their performance is in terms of specific, limited standards which cannot be applied to the more prestigious, higher status "professionals" who counsel clients.

3. Although held accountable for results, they are at the mercy of decisions made by employers who, unlike people with disabilities, are entirely independent of the rehabilitation agency. For the most part, counseling training in the professional patronization of clients is irrelevant when the counselor turns job developer and becomes dependent on the employer.

4. Making matters worse, no reasonable substitute has been found for the title "job developer." The title tends to elicit an indignant and usually inarticulate resentment among business people. Sometimes this attitude is expressed directly: "It is we in business who *develop* the jobs; you people in social agencies only find the ones that we developed."

5. Despite these handicaps, the job developer might manage to scrounge up a modest number of job orders in a local community. Periodically, however, an executive officer of the state agency, whose status provides access to executives of the corporate giants—the telephone company, other public utilities, the auto manufacturers—will influence and thus obtain commitments for hundreds of jobs. Compared with such breakthroughs, the output of the full-time local job developer must seem discouragingly puny.

6. To finish the litany of discontents plaguing the developer, there is no empirically based, organized technology applicable to job development. Everyone either abjures or encourages the job developer, but no one has taken responsibility for developing valid knowledge which could provide tools to do the work.

Given all the problems listed here, not to speak of the intrinsic difficulty of the task, it is possible that even a vast improvement in the technology of job development would contribute relatively little to improving a developer's performance. Still, that possibility can only be tested when the technologies have been developed and used. Therefore, this chapter is addressed to the problem of developing adequate technological systems for job developers.

NEED FOR TASK ANALYSES

As a first step in the development of an empirically based set of technologies for job development, appropriate kinds of task analyses must be made. It is ironic that while job developers are constantly analyzing jobs to isolate skills needed to do work, their own jobs have not been analyzed for the same purpose. To illustrate, Wright and Fraser (1976) identified 14 job placement tasks out of 294 possible tasks of vocational rehabilitation counselors. In a similar study of the specific placement tasks performed by school placement specialists who had other, nonplacement functions, 91 out of a possible 184 *placement-specific* tasks were identified as being frequently performed. These tasks were isolated as above the mean in importance, as the specific responsibility of placement workers (as opposed to counselors and others in placement-related work), and as requiring inservice training in order to be performed effectively. Of those 91 tasks, 40 were specifically concerned with the job development part of the placement process (Gordon et al., in preparation). That is, when the placement role is examined in detail, a good many more than 14 tasks may be identified as essential, even when only the specific job development part of the role is examined.

By and large, previous task analyses have been aimed at building counseling curricula by outlining the major blocks of subject matter to be included in the academic preparation of counselors who may also perform placement functions. Obviously, methods for analyzing tasks are variously useful depending upon purpose. The kind of task analysis suitable for identifying curriculum contents (i.e., cognitive contents) is not particularly useful for developing empirically based technologies (i.e., identification and prescription of performance skills).

There are two kinds of task analysis particularly appropriate for beginning to define job development technologies. The first of these is an assessment of the frequency, importance, and difficulty of performing all of the "complete tasks" in job development. A "complete task" is a statement that systematically fills in all the terms, symbolized by capital letters, in a sentence of the following form:

> A (usually the job developer) does B (a verb of action)
> to C (things, data, or people as objects of the action)
> in D circumstances (when, where, in response to what cues or
>   signals)

in order to achieve E (the immediate objective or output of the task)

as indicated by F (the criteria or cues used to detect whether the goal E was achieved)

with G other possible consequences (unintended or predictable side effects on A, B, C, D, E and/or F).[1]

In a recent study Gordon et al. (in preparation) identified 184 potential tasks performed by school-based job placement specialists in Michigan.[2] Describing each such task in a simplified version of the sentence paradigm (A was not stated, since in all cases it was the job placement specialist, and F and G were omitted) led to the development of a survey instrument which, in turn, was used to determine the reported frequency, importance, and difficulty of each task.

Such an analysis makes it possible to link empirical referents to each of the variables in the task. Thus, the path is set down for developing an empirically based technology for performing the task. Discussion and illustration of how to link a task statement and an empirically based technology occur in later sections of this chapter.

First, however, there is another kind of task analysis that would also be useful to job developers. The survey type described above is generally useful for constructing a picture of the routine or standard features of job development work. However, much of a job developer's success is based not so much on how well routine or standard tasks are handled but rather on how well unexpected, nonstandard, unique, or unpredictable problems are solved. For example, how does the job developer respond to the particular terms in which an employer expresses resistance to hiring a person with a disability? What about the unpredicted consequences of an unsuccessful referral of a client to a job with a "new" employer? How can a particular potential job be made accessible enough so that the job order can be filled? The critical incident technique is particularly useful

---

[1] Although this task statement paradigm appears objective, do not be fooled. The action verb and the objective, like the terms *stimulus* and *response*, may be written at any level of size and complexity. A response unit may be defined to be as small as the action of a single muscle cell or as large as several years of behavior (e.g., "The client's response to the loss of his father was a psychotic episode"). Similarly, there is no way of measuring or specifying the size or complexity of the verb and objective units. For the purpose of linking the elements of a task with empirical knowledge, these terms should be written at the size and complexity levels of the variables frequently studied in social science research, but unfortunately these also vary widely. There is no objective substitute for the experience, knowledge, judgment, and finesse of the task analyst.

[2] The task list was generated through interviews with small groups of job developers which continued until subsequent interviews with new samples yielded no additions to the list. That listing was then submitted to new samples, who screened it for completeness and appropriateness of the vocabulary.

for identifying these nonroutine situations and for describing the performance of job developers in handling them (Flanagan et al., 1949). Again, the results of this kind of task analysis may be expressed systematically through the task sentence paradigm. For example, in one study of job placement workers (paraprofessional placement counselors), incidents were coded and analyzed in terms of the input that triggered an action by the placement worker ("What led up to this incident?"), the objective of the worker (inferred from responses to "How did it turn out?" in successful critical incidents), and the strategies used for each of the objectives associated with a particular input (Gordon and Erfurt, 1973). Thus the outcome of the analysis was in the general form: A did B to C in D circumstances in order to achieve E. It was then possible to identify the frequency with which the various inputs were contained in the sample of critical incidents, and the relative frequencies of the various objectives associated with each class of inputs. For example, for the input "client does not want to accept a referral to a particular job which was consistent with the client's training," the most frequent objective was to convince the client to accept it. When that did not work or was deemed inappropriate, the less frequent objective was to find another job opening more acceptable to the client. Similarly, within each input-objective pair, strategies could be ranked in decreasing order of frequency. Since the critical incident methodology tends to emphasize "critical" or particularly salient tasks, the result is a picture of the performances that are most likely to determine the success of the job placement worker.

LINKING TASKS TO EMPIRICALLY BASED TECHNOLOGIES

The goal of both of the task-analytic studies described above was to produce training materials for job developers. In both cases, the crucial link between the task analysis and the resulting training was absent, as is so often the case in the applied social sciences. That link is the basic, empirical knowledge that would have enabled the designers of the training to say that the job developer *ought* to perform the task or the strategy in a particular way. It must be established that on a particular occasion D, the action term B does lead to the objective E, or that the stimuli described by F are valid indicators of the goal-state. A basis in social science research must be found for converting a *des*criptive task statement into a *pre*scriptive one.

In the absence of that basic step, trainers and educators must fall back on "the accumulated wisdom of the field"—on custom and past usage among experienced job developers and placement workers. That fallback position is not entirely inappropriate. People can be assumed to have learned some things through their experience. Experience is, in a sense, simply a less systematic method of empirical research ("experience" is the French noun, which translates as "experiment" in English). Falling back on past usage and custom does not carry the field forward, however. Experience is conservative. The field needs new methods for solving problems experience has not solved. For example, one recent review of job development models (Johnson, 1978) notes that the standard U.S. Employment Service Handbook on job development instructs the employer relations representative (ERR) to:

1. Use the employer's plan of service to define objectives for the meeting
2. Prepare, by becoming knowledgeable of the employer's operation and needs, the plan of service and employment service capabilities
3. Ensure that individual ERRs conduct their business with those in the firm who have hiring authority
4. Present to the employer the advantage of using the employment service
5. Persuade the employer to discuss his needs
6. Present specific examples of the way the employment service could meet those needs
7. Overcome employer objections
8. Bring the contact with the employer to a clear conclusion
9. Document the visit on the employer record card
10. Perform any follow-up needed

These ideas are so general and time worn that the list is immediately familiar to job developers in schools, vocational rehabilitation (VR), CETA, private employment agencies, indeed, to job developers everywhere. Surely, ways of going beyond citing the standard prescreening of applicants, making available information on applicant skills and performance potential, supplying follow-up support, achieving fast turnaround between receipt of a job order and referral, providing one-stop service, and meeting affirmative action needs must be found. Generating new technologies from concrete research knowledge is a particularly fruitful way to get beyond these traditional and banal methods.

Two approaches to generating empirically based technologies for perfoming job development tasks are presented here. In describing those two approaches, the importance of the systematic form of the task statement paradigm described in the first section of this chapter will become clear.

One approach is to mine the existing empirical literature, largely in psychology, sociology, economics, and their applied versions in counseling, mass communications, and advertising, for extant knowledge concerning each of the variables and their interactions in the A through G task paradigm. For example, one task of a job developer for persons with disabilities might be to convince an employer to hire a client who is marginally below the position requirements in some respect(s). There is voluminous literature concerned with social influence which identifies many of the variables that can change people's attitudes. This literature could be mined for what it implies about characteristics of persuasion or social influence (B in the task paradigm), and which combinations of attributes and techniques influence different kinds of receivers of persuasive communications (C in the task paradigm). There is some literature that points out circumstances under which there is more or less attitudinal and/or behavioral change in response to an influence attempt (D in the task paradigm). Assuming that employers who place job orders with a rehabilitation agency for the first time are adopting an innovation, the growing literature on the diffusion and adoption of innovations in complex organizations could be relevant to job developers. Substituting variables obtained this way for the A through G terms in the task statement, a prescriptive statement can be made.

To take another example: a job developer might have to design a mass mailing to employers in order to increase the number of employer-initiated contacts with the job development office. Relevant to such a task is the vast research on how written stimuli are remembered, on perception, or on associative meanings of words. Information of this sort can be generalized to yield empirically based guidelines for writing an effective circular.

A final example: to encourage a "new" employer to place a job order, job developers frequently employ the tactic of telling about an employer who has successfully hired people with disabilities. A substantial body of research exists on modeling, imitation, and self-other comparisons that could be tapped for principles that could guide the job developer in deciding which employers to cite to which prospects. Some research suggests that people tend to compare themselves moderately upward—that is, they tend to imitate models who are *moderately* but not greatly above them in such things as skill, status, or success. Thus, one would cite a moderately larger machine shop to a small parts manufacturer, but forego using a corporate giant as an example.

The second approach for linking research knowledge to job development tasks in order to generate a valid technology is one that takes a more direct path. When tasks are stated in a systematic form, it is possible to identify successful and unsuccessful performances. In the paradigm, that means performances or enactments of a particular task that do and those that do not achieve their intended objective. Performances can then be compared on each of the other variables in the paradigm: attributes of successful and unsuccessful performers, comparisons of the kinds of actions taken, attributes of the recipients of the actions, and so on. At a more gross level, more versus less successful job developers could be identified by criteria based on dollar value, in wages, of job orders generated per time period. These two groups could then be compared for both the frequency with which they perform the tasks and to determine the main variables within each complete task statement. In the study of school-based job placement specialists, it was found that "exemplary" incumbents differed from the others by performing various public relations tasks more frequently and placing less importance on tasks involving direct interactions with clients seeking referrals to jobs. The study did not go beyond that level of analysis, but it would be feasible to compare these exemplaries with non-exemplaries on such matters as how they go about performing each of the tasks. Such comparisons could then yield a set of sentences, in task-specific terms, specifying optimum technologies for job developers to use, given the present state of the art.

There are risks of misinformation in each of these two approaches. Indeed, there is no foolproof method for bridging the gap between empirical descriptive statements (e.g., that one variant of A produces more or less B than another variant of A) and empirically based prescriptive statements (e.g., that job developers *should* have this attribute in order to do B). Still, each of the two approaches risks a different kind of error. Because of that, they can check on each others' effectiveness in solving a given problem.

The major point is that task analyses made in the form recommended in this chapter identify task variables that can be associated with the variables studied in social science research. They can also be associated with the performances of successful and unsuccessful job developers, thus facilitating the application of research knowledge to the development of valid job development technologies.

MAJOR JOB DEVELOPMENT
TASKS AND SOME EMPIRICAL REFERENTS

The remainder of this chapter will illustrate some of the earlier points by describing some of the job development tasks that might emerge from the recommended task analyses and some kinds of social science research that could be mined in order to generate the relevant technologies.

Table 1 lists the job development tasks that emerged as high-priority tasks of school-based job placement specialists. These are the tasks that a sample of 181 respondents said they performed frequently, that is, above the mean on frequency for all 184 tasks in the inventory. They were rated above the mean for all tasks in ascribed importance, and were above the mean in felt need for inservice training. Fifty percent or more of the

Table 1. Priority job development tasks of school-based job placement specialists in Michigan

Tasks	Exemplaries
1. Decide how to make an initial contact with a potential employer.	
2. Plan and conduct surveys of employers in the community to assess hiring needs, job qualifications, working conditions, willingness to hire students, and interest in use of the school placement service.	H
3. Identify a prospective employer's employment needs that you could meet as a way of providing services and developing a good relationship which would result in job orders.	H
4. Identify and use contacts in the business community and in civic organizations to facilitate contacts with employers and their use of the school placement program.	H
5. Explain to an employer the contents of various school courses and the skills acquired in them as they relate to a job, entry or skill requirements, hiring standards, or personnel assignment.	H
6. Convince an employer to list job openings with the school placement service.	
7. Find out who the appropriate persons are to contact in a prospective employing organization.	
8. Find out which employers in the community have current job openings for which students might qualify.	
9. Find out from trade or business associations or from informal employer networks which employers are likely to be hiring in the future in jobs for which students might qualify.	H
10. Find out from an employer what job openings he has, hiring standards and job qualifications, work requirements, pay, work conditions, fringe benefits, career or advancement ladders, and relevant personnel policies.	
11. Respond effectively to an employer's negative attitude toward the school, its students, or programs.	H
12. Provide student records and information to prospective employers without violating confidentiality rules and laws.	
13. Contact an employer to tell him that you cannot fill a particular job order.	
14. Obtain all relevant information when taking a job order.	
15. Explain to employers child labor laws, minimum wage requirements, and/or equal opportunity requirements regarding minorities, women, and the handicapped.	
16. Prepare and deliver speeches and/or other presentations to community or other nonschool groups.	H
17. Assess a job opening with regard to the requirements of child labor and minimum wage laws.	

Table 1—*continued*

	Tasks	Exemplaries
18.	Plan a public relations or information campaign to facilitate or increase use of the job placement program and/or the successful employment of students.	
19.	Manage the writing of copy and the design of art work for placement promotional materials.	
20.	Write press releases and get them used by the media.	H
21.	Gain the support or interest of local media for free or low cost publicity.	H
22.	Make contact with a student's immediate supervisor to follow up on a placement, identify problems, help resolve problems, and/or get early information about potential job openings.	
23.	Provide feedback to counselors and vocational and other teachers on the placement outcomes of particular students.	
24.	Identify curriculum revisions to improve the employability of students.	H
25.	Convince teachers and/or administrators to introduce curriculum revisions designed to improve student employability.	
26.	Provide labor market information to school staff in a way that would make it useful in teaching, counseling, and curriculum planning.	H
27.	Help other school staff develop materials for teaching pre-employment skills.	
28.	Initiate, plan, or present inservice training relevant to job placement to school staff.	H
29.	Identify the population to be served by the placement program.	
30.	Operate a clearinghouse for part-time and after-school hours jobs.	
31.	Draft proposals for funds for placement program innovations and seek support for the proposals.	H
32.	Maintain and make available for use by students and/or staff a file of occupational information or information resources.	
33.	Maintain a system for receiving and recording job orders from employers.	
34.	Establish and maintain a system for routing job orders to staff and students who might fill the orders.	
35.	Monitor and follow up on job orders to see that they are filled promptly.	
36.	Design forms and establish and maintain a records system for keeping track of placement services and activities.	
37.	Design and conduct systematic follow-up of placements by questioning employers and/or students on	

continued

Table 1—*continued*

Tasks	Exemplaries
job retention, promotions, wages, sources of difficulty, and/or satisfaction.	
38. Maintain, update, and make available for use by students and/or staff a file on local employers, their entry level jobs, employment requirements, and other relevant information.	
39. Establish a system to monitor and coordinate job development contacts to avoid duplication of effort or failure to follow through in a timely manner.	
40. Analyze and summarize follow-up, employer and/or student survey data, and write reports.	

respondents said these tasks were primarily the responsibility of the job placement program as compared with counselors, administrators, and vocational and other teachers. The sample was subdivided into full-time, part-time, and placement program directors; when a task met at least 75% of the criteria for each of the subgroups, it was identified as a high-priority task, and from that group, those that are intrinsic to job development were selected for this listing.[3] Those tasks that were significantly higher ($p < 0.05$) in rating of importance or frequency of performance by a subgroup of 14 exemplary placement specialists, when compared with non-exemplary full-time placement specialists, are indicated by H; those on which the exemplaries were significantly lower ($p < 0.05$) are indicated by L.

Table 2 lists those tasks of the placement specialists that did not meet the criteria for Table 1, but on which the exemplary specialists differed significantly from the non-exemplaries ($p \leq 0.05$). Again, H and L are used to identify the direction of the difference.

Table 2 suggests that exemplary placement specialists put more emphasis on links with the community, collecting and managing objective information, particularly providing labor market information to teachers, and high visibility activities. Less emphasis was placed on addressing specific needs of individual candidates for job placement.

Table 3 illustrates the kinds of tasks that might emerge from use of the critical incident technique. The table summarizes the findings of a study of paraprofessional placement workers in a Chicago anti-poverty agency concerned with placing people from minority groups in jobs. This agency operated on the "hire now and train later" principle. Each respondent was responsible for a specific list of employers with whom the

---

[3] I have included in this listing not only the tasks that have as their immediate objective the generation of job orders, but also those linkage tasks, which those who do job development carry out in support of their job development activities.

Table 2.   Tasks on which exemplary placement specialists differ from non-exemplaries

Tasks	Exemplaries
1. Obtain statistics that show the employability, placement potential, and/or advantages of hiring students through your program, and put them in a form to display to prospective employers.	H
2. Obtain information from local unions about job openings and occupational requirements, help in getting job orders, or participation in special projects (job fair, job familiarization).	H
3. Provide information to appropriate community organizations to help them convince an employer to relocate into your community.	H
4. Inform an employer about alternative forms of personnel utilization (e.g., flexi-time, shared jobs).	H
5. Develop and coordinate plans with local government officials regarding industrial development for expanded employment.	H
6. Plan and prepare a periodic newsletter for distribution to students, staff, parents, community, and/or employers.	H
7. Explain to students what worker's compensation is and eligibility for benefits.	L
8. Teach or advise students about dress and grooming for job-searching, applying, and working.	L
9. Explain to students the eligibility requirements for unemployment compensation and how to apply for it.	L
10. Help students identify their career goals and make specific career plans.	H
11. Make arrangements for placement staff and vocational or other teachers to tour employment sites where students have been or may be placed.	H
12. Arrange for the school to provide a special training program to meet an employer's need.	H
13. Prompt teachers to include pre-employment and placement concepts and skills as topics for class or as homework assignments.	H
14. Provide student information to other community agencies without violating confidentiality rules and laws.	L
15. Plan, conduct, supervise, or organize activities such as a job fair or a career day.	H
16. Develop and implement joint planning and programs with coop education; special needs; special education; vocational education, guidance, and counseling; and/or other work experience or employment preparation programs within the school or school system.	H
17. Assist in planning and conducting placement program staff meetings.	H

continued

Table 2—*continued*

Tasks	Exemplaries
18. Decide on membership of a placement advisory committee and obtain their participation.	H
19. Establish the roles and functions of a placement advisory committee and communicate them to the committee.	H
20. Participate in setting agendas, scheduling meetings, and conducting placement advisory committee meetings.	H
21. Identify placement program policy options and assist placement advisory committee to make policy recommendations.	H
22. Explain job placement programs and activities and make presentations to the placement advisory committee.	H
23. Facilitate cooperative interaction within the placement advisory committee and between the committee and the program or school.	H

agency had relationships and for placing clients with those employers. The column headings in the table refer to the main elements of the systematic task paradigm. Thus, the first column describes the input circumstance (D) that initiated an activity by the respondent, the second column summarizes the objectives (E) served by the activity, and the third column summarizes the techniques used (i.e., the action B, and the object of the action C). The last column summarizes the organizational structure, supports, and resources that facilitate performance of the task. The first row of the table summarizes these task variables for the most frequent input reported in the critical incidents, the second row the next most frequent input, and so on. Within the Objective and Strategies cells, items are listed in order of frequency.

What is necessary now is to illustrate how the tasks described in the three tables may be linked with empirically based knowledge in order to provide technologies that will help perform them effectively. Research literature on the diffusion and adoption of innovations has been selected as one source of information particularly pertinent to many of the job development tasks listed. Literature on attitude formation and change, interpersonal influence, social power and influence, behavior change processes, decision-making, personnel utilization, persuasion, and interviewing techniques, among other possibilities, would also be relevant.

Generalizations from the innovation diffusion and adoption literature have been made largely based on the reviews by Rogers and Shoemaker (1971), Zaltman, Duncan, and Holbek (1973), and Rothman

Table 3. Critical tasks of placement workers

Problems	Objectives	Strategies	Resources
1. Enrollee needs a job or training placement.	To place the enrollee on a job or in training.	1. Search for a slot that fits the enrollee's bill. 2. Get enrollee to accept an available opening. 3. Prepare enrollee so he looks good to employer. 4. Intervene with employer so he will accept enrollee. 5. Get both enrollee and employer to make some changes.	1. An employer intelligence system. 2. Access to legal expertise. 3. Job search workshop. 4. Effective team structure.
2. Enrollee rejects job referral.	A. Convince enrollee to take the first referral. B. Find another placement.	1. One-to-one counseling. 2. Persuasion. 3. Prove sincerity and commitment. 4. Change the referral.	1. Feedback, supervision, and appropriate evaluation. 2. Organizational consensus. 3. Access to job orders. 4. Grievance machinery for enrollees. 5. Status of minorities and coaches within the agency.

continued

Table 3—*continued*

	Problems		Objectives		Strategies		Resources
3.	Uncooperative or resistant employer.		Get company to hire and retain minority employees.	1.	Get company involved in agency's program.	1.	Planning for employer involvement.
				2.	Arrange a successful experience for the employer.	2.	Employer follow-up.
						3.	Employer relations and job development strategies.
				3.	Get company to change its people.		
				4.	Become legalistic.	4.	Training in equal opportunity law.
4.	Enrollee has been fired or laid off.		Keep the enrollee on the job.	1.	Check out nature of the problem.	1.	Racial/ethnic staff mixture.
				2.	Negotiate with the company.	2.	Flexible orientation.
				3.	Negotiate with the enrollee.	3.	Access to employer.
						4.	Access to supportive service.
				4.	Make a plan and carry it out.	5.	Adequate records.
5.	Enrollee quitting the job.	A.	Keep the enrollee on the job.	1.	Help him achieve incentives.	1.	Long-term relationship with employers.
		B.	Get the enrollee a different placement.	2.	Show the disadvantages of quitting.	2.	Technical expertise in job description and performance standards.
		C.	Prevent the spread of dissatisfaction.	3.	Encourage enrollee to stay at job until something better turns up.		
				4.	Help him with personal problems.	3.	Relationships with enrollees' families.
				5.	Refer enrollee to a different job.	4.	Flexibility in working with enrollees.
						5.	Criteria for judging success of coaching.
				6.	Take enrollee out of the job market.	6.	Suitable schools for dropouts and adults.

6. Enrollee in trouble with the law.	A. Free the enrollee. B. Save the enrollee's job.	1. Advocate for the enrollee to the court. 2. Give evidence for the enrollee. 3. Get legal resources. 4. Get the charges dropped. 5. Give emotional support to the enrollee. 6. Advocate to the employer. 7. Line up a job for after jail.	1. Inservice legal training. 2. Specialized court unit. 3. Linkages to sources of legal aid.
7. Enrollee's personal welfare in danger.	Promote enrollee's health and welfare.	1. Advise the enrollee. 2. Change the enrollee's experience. 3. Act for the enrollee.	1. Mental health consultation. 2. Access to drug treatment programs.

From Gordon and Erfurt (1973) by permission.

(1974). Derived from these generalizations, various techniques are listed that could be used to perform many of the job development tasks summarized in the tables. Underlying this presentation is the assumption that getting an employer to offer jobs to people who are different from other employees—that is, to a person with a disability or to people referred from an agency that the employer never used before, is a case of trying to get the employer to adopt an innovation. An organization is more likely to adopt an innovation if:

1. The innovation can be tried out on a small scale.
    a. Hire a client for a short, fixed period, such as a month, as a trial.
    b. Hire a client part-time at first.
    c. Try one client to see how it works out before agreeing to place job orders routinely.
    d. Hire a client in one special section of the employing establishment in which failure risks, as seen by the employer, have low associated costs.
2. The innovation can be reversed if it does not work out.
    a. Fill temporary short-term personnel needs at first for a first trial of hiring workers through the program.
    b. Reduce the costs of laying off or firing a client who does not work out by informing the employer that the agency will continue to work with the client and the employer.
    c. Make the client's first assignment to a unit of the employer's company in which there is a rapid rate of transfer of personnel into and out of the unit.
    d. Inform the employer of second-injury legislation and protections against an increase in the employer's experience rating for unemployment compensation contributions.
3. The innovation is not too different from what the organization has done in the past or is now doing.
    a. Describe the placement program as an improvement in effectiveness, not as a pioneering or radically new system.
    b. Use the employer's language, concepts, and values in describing the placement service and its clients.
    c. Make proposals to employers in such a way as to make them seem consistent with the employer's usual or preferred ways of doing things.
    d. Justify use of the placement program through reference to the employer's values, philosophy, and business and personal principles rather than attempt to change the employer's assumptions, prejudices, or perceptions.

e. Stress the similarities between the program's clients and those hired in the past through the employer's usual sources.

f. Identify the similarity in educational background and previous work experience of placement program clients with those presently employed in the firm, with employees already on the payroll who have disabilities, or with employees who became impaired, even temporarily, through illness or accident, and who continued their employment.

g. Compare clients with limited education with employees hired in the past, when limited education was more frequent than it is today.

h. Describe any special employer service, such as work station modification or a special orientation to the job, as small extensions of what the employer already does.

4. The innovation is accepted and used by others with whom the employer compares himself.

a. Cite employers in the same or similar industry who enjoy the same or slightly better success in terms of size, prestige, or profitability and who use the placement service.

b. Identify previous employers of the client who are similar to the prospective employer.

c. Cite business people with similar or slightly higher prestige who are related to the placement program or the agency as members of boards or advisory committees, who have provided advice to the agency or performed some service for it such as donating equipment, or who have served as volunteer "big brothers" to clients regarding their vocational choice and preparation.

d. Put leaders of trade, industry, and merchants' associations on advisory committees and give them serious tasks to perform to keep them involved and publicly committed to the agency and its program.

e. Provide opportunities for business people to serve as spokespersons for the program in public meetings and media.

f. Describe the agency or program in order to emphasize its relationship to industry and the market rather than its relationship to government sponsorship, funds, or public welfare programs.

5. The employer hears about the innovation from local opinion leaders whose judgment he respects.

a. Arrange for opportunities for members of local associations of business people, personnel managers, engineers, and trade and professional associations to talk to each other about their experience in hiring clients through the placement program, or clients similar to those served by the agency.

    b.   Use someone of comparable status to the employer and known to the employer as an intermediary in setting up the first contact and/or to be present during the first contact to describe a good experience with the placement agency.

    c.   Use mass media to create a good climate of opinion in the employer's business or residential community, stressing that it is normal to hire clients like those served by the placement program, not a special, extraordinary, or risky act.

    d.   In using mass media, make it seem routine that clients thought to have a disability in fact perform well, rather than emphasizing the extraordinary drive or unusual talent of an exceptional client.

    e.   Cite the large number of employers who use the placement service rather than a single unusual or outstanding employer.

6.   There is little or no uncertainty about the innovation.

    a.   Spell out exactly what the client can do as an employee, the specific machines that the individual can operate, and so on.

    b.   Start with minimal risk clients and escalate the risks as confidence grows.

    c.   Be specific and clear about how the employer is to transmit job orders, how soon a referral will be made, and how frequently and when follow-up will occur.

7.   Organizational gatekeepers accept the innovation.

    a.   Identify gaps between decisions made by top management and those made at lower levels that affect the hiring process.

    b.   If foremen or shop supervisors have the right to accept or reject a job applicant, either informally or formally, make a persuasive presentation to them.

    c.   Have the employer assign the first hires through the placement program to those supervisors with the most prestige with other supervisors in the company.

    d.   If there are concerns about how present employees would react to the client's uniqueness, offer to meet those who would be in closest contact with the client. They might fear the possibility that they would have to increase their own productivity to compensate for low productivity they expect from the client.

8.   The costs of the innovation (e.g., time, money, effort) are less than the costs of other alternatives.

    a.   Minimize the employer's start-up or first-time costs by making contacts with the employer brief and crisp, minimizing the employer's paper work in connection with the transaction, referring carefully screened clients, reducing needs to place want ads and then interviewing large numbers of people. Provide dollar estimates of cost savings.

b. Help the employer meet affirmative action requirements before the company has to contend with charges and investigations.

c. Provide the employer with referral help to community agencies for "troubled employees."

d. When a particular job order cannot be filled by the placement program, check other agencies on behalf of the employer to save the employer from having to replace the job order elsewhere.

9. The employer is a high technology company involved in, say, electronics, advanced engineering, or manufacture of medical instruments with diversified jobs, a professional staff, and employees who travel widely to professional meetings, trade shows, and business meetings.

a. Give highest priority to job development contacts with companies of this type, which are most likely to adopt innovations, influence others, and accept social responsibilities.

b. Use these kinds of companies to influence their suppliers and other more "local" kinds of employers to use the placement service.

10. There is visible evidence of the effectiveness of the innovation.

a. Use a portfolio with graphic presentations of statistics on such matters as median wages of clients placed by the program, job-loss or quit-rate of clients, and other productivity measures.

b. Similar data from the research literature on programs and clients like those of the placement agency should also be displayed in graphic form.

c. Include photographs of successfully placed clients at their work stations. Use action-pictures of the clients at work with complicated-looking equipment and label the photos with brief client and employer data.

11. Attitude formation is followed by a decision, which is then implemented.

a. Attach a specific, agreed-upon action step to each commitment or decision made by the employer.

b. Follow up on oral agreements with a letter that states the decision that has been reached, who will do what next, and when.

c. Propose specific implementation steps, with suggested times, for each verbal agreement reached.

d. Offer to assist with implementation steps, or provide models of such steps. An example of a memo used by another employer for informing the personnel office about the agreement to place job orders with the placement agency is such a model.

No doubt other action guidelines could be drawn from these generalizations about the adoption of innovations in complex organizations, and, of course, not all of these can be used successfully in every circumstance. Nevertheless, the possibilities outlined here do support the belief that the empirical social science literature can be mined for information that can suggest strategies and techniques for accomplishing the tasks of job developers in new and effective ways.

SUMMARY

It is not clear that even perfect use of job development techniques can contribute much improvement to the effectiveness of placement programs, given the organizational factors that affect job developers' work. However, until such a body of empirically based techniques has been developed, the relative contributions of market forces, structural constraints, and the like cannot be assessed.

In order to develop a technology for job development, the tasks performed by job developers should be systematically analyzed so that the task elements can be connected with the variables studied in social science research. A paradigm for describing tasks in such terms was presented along with two methodologies for performing the analyses and organizing the data.

The next step is to link the tasks with empirical knowledge. One way to do that is to mine the existing social science literature for relationships among variables such as those contained in the task statements. This way, task descriptions can be converted into prescriptive statements. Another idea is to use a "best practices" approach, in which the techniques used by more successful job developers in the performance of each task are identified.

Finally, illustrative material from studies of job placement workers were used to suggest the kinds of job development tasks that are performed and how many of these tasks can be linked with an empirical base. For purposes of this illustration, the social science reasearch in innovation diffusion and adoption in complex organizations was reviewed and some relevant generalizations made. These were then applied by listing job development techniques that are consistent with the generalizations derived from the literature and relevant to many of the tasks identified.

REFERENCES

Flanagan, J., et al. 1949. Critical Requirements for Research Personnel. American Institute for Research, Pittsburgh.

Fraser, R. T., and Wright, G. N. 1977. Improving rehabilitation personnel managment. J. Rehab. 43(3):22–24.

Gordon, J., Anderson, C., Martin, J., and Young, W. Job placement specialists' tasks and training needs: A survey. In preparation.

Gordon, J., and Erfurt, J. 1973. Placement and After: A Manual for Coaches and Other Employment Workers. Institute of Labor and Industrial Relations, Ann Arbor, Michigan.

Johnson, M. 1978. Job Development and Placement: CETA Program Models. U.S. Government Printing Office, Washington, D.C.

Rogers, E., and Shoemaker, F. 1971. Communication of Innovations. Free Press, New York.

Rothman, J. 1974. Planning and Organizing for Community Change. Columbia University Press, New York.

Wright, G. N., and Fraser, R. T. 1976. Improving Manpower Utilization: The Rehabilitation Task Performance Evaluation Scale. University of Wisconsin Rehabilitation Research Institute, Wisconsin Studies in Vocational Rehabilitation, Madison.

Zaltman, G., Duncan, R., and Holbek, J. 1973. Innovations and Organizations. John Wiley & Sons, Inc., New York.

Chapter 7

Job Analysis in Vocational Rehabilitation

James Engelkes

Editor's note: Job analysis has been a traditional but often neglected tool of rehabilitation counselors and placement specialists. The process is not unique to rehabilitation, but evolved in an industrial context, as this chapter points out. One possible reason for neglect is that the purposes and methods of analyzing jobs have been borrowed too directly from industry and have not been adapted for rehabilitation uses. This chapter seeks to provide a way of using job analysis from a rehabilitation perspective.

This chapter shows how job analysis can be specifically related to many activities within the rehabilitation process. When used properly, a job analysis permits a counselor and client to put the information obtained about the client from evaluation into a world-of-work context. This process can provide systematic direction for planning appropriate change strategies. It also helps the counselor ensure that rehabilitation services in general remain relevant to the local labor market. This chapter also stresses that job analysis, when used to plan for job restructuring, can provide counselors and employers with an opportunity to collaborate in developing advancement opportunites, thus contributing to the career enhancement of persons with disabilities.

Job analysis has other implications for relationships with employers. Conducting a systematic job analysis shows an employer that a rehabilitation professional is a vocational expert who will provide a valuable, relevant, and job-ready pool of applicants. Job analysis can be a job development tool and an activity that strengthens the tie between employers and rehabilitation professionals.

This chapter provides further evidence of the value of viewing the rehabilitation professional's role as an information broker. Job analyses provide important information for individual clients that helps them make choices about vocational directions. Job analyses provide counselors with up-to-date information about the labor market and are a vehicle for developing relationships with employers. All of this information can be fed back into the rehabilitation system to help it remain responsive to the business community, thus helping rehabilitation fulfill its vocational obligations to its clientele.

In addition, this chapter presents two illustrations of job analysis procedures. These have been developed for the busy rehabilitation practitioner who has heavy caseload requirements. These forms show how brief analyses can eliminate unnecessary analytical work and help the professional focus on issues most important for facilitating the successful rehabilitation of a particular client. As a supplement to this chapter, specific training in the technical aspects of conducting extensive job analysis is recommended.

—

Since the passage of the rehabilitation legislation of 1973 and 1974, practitioners in the field of rehabilitation have focused their attention on persons with severe impairments. Generally, these people suffer from serious work disabilities. Under prior legislation, people with severe disabilities were often rejected for services because it was assumed that they would insufficiently respond to rehabilitation. The severity of a given physical or mental impairment itself seemed to cause this problem. However, research has found that the functional limitations resulting from an impairment, rather than the impairment itself, are important in determining the extent of work disability. Other factors, such as age and extent of education, also mediate the degree of work disability. The rehabilitation community is now required to prepare people with severe disabilities for competitive employment. It is true that the number of rehabilitations achieved by the state/federal system has declined for the first time in many years. This has probably been the result of a change in caseload composition. However, it has also been shown that many people with severe disabilities have achieved successful competitive employment. One of the old rehabilitation tools, job analysis, has had continuous value in the rehabilitation of these persons, since it is a tool that focuses on specific functions required to do a certain job. This chapter reviews the concept of job analysis and suggests how it can be used effectively in rehabilitation.

In today's society, the word *job* has different meanings depending on how, when, or by whom it is used. The words *job, position, task,* and *career* have become almost interchangeable. Some of the confusion regarding these terms has been eliminated for the professional rehabilitation practitioner through definitions provided by the U.S. Training and Employment Service:

1. *Element* is the smallest step into which it is practical to subdivide any work activity without analyzing separate motions, movements, and mental processes involved.
2. *Task* is one or more elements and is one of the distinct activities that constitute logical and necessary steps in the performance of work by the worker. A task is created whenever human effort, physical or mental, is exerted to accomplish a specific purpose.
3. *Position* is a collection of tasks constituting the total work assignment of a single worker. There are as many positions as there are workers in the country.
4. *Job* is a group of positions that are identical with respect to their major or significant tasks and sufficiently alike to justify their being covered by a single analysis. There may be one or many persons

employed in the same job (United States Department of Labor, 1972).

Additional definitions that will also keep terminology clear are:

Occupation is gainfully employed activity and is made up of a group of similar jobs which may be found from situation to situation.

Career is a total composite of one's activities throughout life.

Vocation originates from a Greek word meaning a "calling." It is frequently used synonymously with the term *career* (Norris et al., 1979).

"Job information is the basic data used by industry, governmental and private agencies, and employee organizations for many manpower programs. The nature of the required job information varies in type and approach according to program needs. Regardless of the ultimate use for which it is intended, however, the data must be accurate; inclusive, omitting nothing pertinent to the program; and presented in a form suitable for study and use. The techniques for obtaining and presenting this information are known as 'job analysis'" (United States Department of Labor, 1972). According to this concept, job analysis can be broadly defined as a systematic attempt to collect and synthesize any information about jobs.

WHAT IS JOB ANALYSIS?

Job analysis is an organized, intensive, and direct method of obtaining the pertinent facts about jobs. The process involves an understanding of the job, which includes material obtained through personal observation or in conversation with workers, supervisors, and others who have information of value. Job analysis is a basic method of gathering information widely accepted throughout industry. It is also used extensively by both military and civilian government. When only one position is involved in the report, the term *position analysis* is used. However, the job, which by definition includes several similar positions, is more frequently the unit of study.

Although the distinction is often a subtle one, job analysis should be differentiated from worker analysis. In worker analysis, the workers performing jobs are studied rather than the tasks. The investigation may be conducted by interviewing, testing, or examining workers. In job analysis, workers are observed, but emphasis is on work activity rather than on their characteristics as individuals. It is true that studies of workers yield information that is helpful in understanding jobs, but job analysis as used in this chapter refers to the process of observing such things as duties involved in jobs, obtaining facts about qualifications required, and collecting other data about the job itself. It is also important for the counselor to assess the individual who is being considered for employment. Conducting a job analysis of an individual's vocational objectives provides information for a comparison between that person's abilities and the requirements of a job.

Occasionally a person who is studying a job intensively will actually do the work to get the "feel" of the job. Also, some analyses involve time and motion study and are made by trained industrial engineers.

The specific technique for conducting a job analysis is straightforward and need not be explicated at this point. See "Job Analysis in Vocational Rehabilitation" (Engelkes, 1978) for a step-by-step procedure to follow when conducting a job analysis. Another helpful guide is the United States Department of Labor's *Handbook for Analyzing Jobs* (1972).

HISTORICAL PERSPECTIVE

Job analysis was originated by industrial engineers, efficiency experts, and industrial managers. Frederick Taylor formally began studying work in the late 1800s with a systematic and scientific approach that viewed individuals in a mechanistic way, with no reference to the psychological and social influences that might affect their work. Taylor divided tasks into units of motion to determine the efficient methods of accomplishing tasks (Nadler, 1963).

"The qualitative analysis of work, encompassing the human element, was initiated by Frank and Lillian Gilbreth. Their concepts of psychology and human relationships affecting work behavior added dimension to Taylor's work. Job analysis was further expanded in the 1950's and applied to personnel psychology, and the study and application of work assessment techniques to improve employee selection" (Bowman and Graves, 1976).

A need exists, then, to combine the kind of objectivity achieved from a mechanistic approach with the human aspects of analysis to gain an accurate and utilitarian understanding of a job. Rehabilitation counselors must assess mechanistic information about jobs in order to apply it to the cases of people with disabilities who can obtain employment given training, job modification or restructuring, counseling, or through other adaptations, whether personal or related to the work setting. Human and mechanistic aspects of analysis must both be considered in order to help persons with disabilities, counselors, rehabilitation programs, employers, and communities through successful placement (Mallik and Sablowsky, 1975).

JOB ANALYSIS IN REHABILITATION TODAY

Basically there are only three parts to the analysis of any job. First, the job itself must be identified completely and accurately. Second, the tasks of the job must be described completely and accurately. Finally, the requirements the job makes upon the worker for successful performance must be indicated.

Any further considerations involve specific programs and have specified uses. The second part of the analysis, the complete and accurate description of the job tasks, is crucial. If this requirement remains unfulfilled, the rest of the analysis is useless.

All counselors who make placements use job analysis information, whether they refer to it as such or not. This information should be gathered systematically and placed on file permanently. A careful job analysis, even if it was made originally for a specific person, will be useful time and again.

Consider for a moment the purpose of a job analysis. By obtaining information from an employer, supervisor, personnel worker, or from all of these people, the counselor has concrete information about a job. The act of obtaining job descriptions is useful in itself; the rehabilitation professional must observe an employee actually performing the job being analyzed. By doing that, the counselor acquires an understanding about that job that goes beyond what can be learned from merely hearing or reading about it. The rehabilitation professional's knowledge about a particular job can be extended to include other, similar jobs in business and industry. Thus, the counselor is able to make judgments and help individuals decide whether their capabilities are appropriate for specific jobs. With sufficient information at hand, the rehabilitation professional is able to intelligently engage in the processes of differential job selection. This is the essential purpose of job analysis. It is also necessary to recognize that informal and formal means can be used to conduct a job analysis. Formal checklists have been developed to guide the actual observation of a job. Obtaining job descriptions, as mentioned, is another formal means. Informal discussions with employers and job holders also provide valuable information and should not be neglected.

The person receiving rehabilitation services brings a composite of cognitive, emotive, and psychomotor skills, along with a set of attitudes, beliefs, and personality traits, to the counselor. It becomes the responsibility of the rehabilitation professional to assess a person's attributes so that recommendations can be made regarding vocational goals and potential training that will help the person become more compatible with the requirements employers have for job applicants. Each person has a number of attributes that could be incorporated into a variety of positions in a variety of jobs. The counselor's purpose is to facilitate the person's job search so that the applicant, as well as potential employers, understands the range of possibilities inherent in the unique set of attributes that person brings to work.

A number of assessment devices evaluate an individual's attributes as they presently exist and help develop techniques for changing these attributes to increase a client's marketability. Typical kinds of assessment would include medical examination and related specialist evaluations; psychological evaluations focusing upon intellectual, emotional, and vocational functioning; and vocational evaluation including structured evaluation procedures, work samples, work attitudes, work behaviors, personal grooming skills, and interpersonal relationship skills. Especially for individuals with severe disabilities, a comprehensive evaluation must be considered before the job-search process can begin. How can rehabilitation professionals and the people they serve proceed with a job search unless the strengths and weakness of each individual are clear? How can rehabilitation professionals assist people in job searches without a comprehensive knowledge of work sites, architectural accessibility, transportation options to and from the work site, job descriptions, compensation and fringe benefits, design of the specific work area, coworker and supervisory attitudes toward people with disabilities, and the current and projected need for the unique skills that a person has to offer?

Rehabilitation professionals have an obligation to fully understand the people they serve just as they must be acquainted with the local labor market. That way, accurate and usable data regarding both can be synthesized and people can be guided into the best work situation available at the time.

THE USES OF JOB ANALYSIS

Rehabilitation professionals may be viewed as consultants who choreograph the job-search process. The job-search process is that activity designed to ensure that a person's skills are used as fully as possible at the best possible wage (where wage includes benefits and job conditions), given the costs of job search and the state of the labor market (Vandergoot, Jacobsen, and Worrall, this volume). It is important to note that the consultant may act on behalf of an individual and is not constrained to working only through the individual. This occurs if the consultant finds it necessary to intervene for a person at certain points in the job-search process.

Two other concepts that involve the use of job analysis information include human engineering and job engineering or modification. When providing services, rehabilitation professionals must be concerned about personal modifications that could help individuals perform the functions of their jobs to the best of their abilities. Would it help a person to perform a particular job if different orthotic or prosthetic devices were tried? If an individual's capabilities can be increased through human engineering so that the person's work tolerance, range of motion, speed, or transfer from one task site to another is improved, then the concepts of human engineering have been applied to make the individual better able to meet the demands of a job. If human engineering principles cannot solve the problems that stand between a person and a job, then the concept of job engineering or modification can be considered. Here the focus is on adapting the job to conform to the individual. The height and slope of a work bench may be redesigned. A different seat may be used, or a microfiche reader with foot controls might be substituted for a telephone directory. These are examples of job engineering that change the job itself, to a greater or lesser degree, so that it can be performed by a certain person.

Implicit to the understanding of human or job engineering is an underlying knowledge of individual attributes and possible human adaptations to given situations. This information can be combined with job analysis and possible job modifications which, if adopted, would aid in the placement of an otherwise hard-to-place individual. This leads to the collection of data that seem applicable only to a single job-seeker. Therefore job analysis, to some counselors, seems to be a time-consuming activity that hinders proper coordination of services. However, if job analysis is viewed broadly as a technique for accumulating information about work in general, then it becomes a resource of information available to everyone involved in a job search. For example, information regarding the recruitment practices of firms can be used to plan individual job searches. This information would also help in the creation of broad-based approaches to changing discriminatory hiring practices.

The counselor can learn a great deal by studying job analysis files, such as whether a company simply hires employees off the street, or whether it works with the state employment service or private employment services, or whether the company's personnel department has a specific screening procedure for specific types of potential employees. This sort of material can help the counselor aid individuals by providing information regarding families of jobs in the community that may be accessible to them. Recognizing that information has both specific and general uses might also reduce the fear that job analysis is too time consuming.

Two questions might be of interest. How do industries view a counselor coming in to do a job analysis? Would it be necessary to make a new job analysis each time a specific person is considered for a specific job in a particular industrial setting? In response to the first question, the company official is usually quick to give information if the rehabilitation professional is clearly a potential aid in the selection of new employees. The second question can be answered briefly by stating that the analysis of the job will remain the same regardless of the nature of the potential employee being considered for it. Again, job analysis is not a worker analysis but defines the specific operations and responsibilities of a specific job. Therefore, one job analysis on each specific job will suffice as long as the job remains the same, that is, until modifications are made regarding job responsibilities or organizational structure.

What other contributions can job analysis make in vocational placement? A frequent reason for job quits or firing is a failure to consider the variables of a job before placement. Social and psychological factors important for work adjustment are sometimes overlooked, even within a systematic analysis. A written job analysis is of aid to the extent that it ensures that a rehabilitation professional will not forget to gather information on some of these important variables. Written analysis also helps the counselor avoid repetitive or intrusive contacts with employers or personnel officers for information that has been given once already.

Job analysis information, as described here, can be useful and dependable because it is likely to be complete and well structured. A library of job analysis may be considered as a systematic attempt to organize knowledge about the various jobs in the community. The abbreviated job analysis form, included here as Table 1, involves little information about a specific job, but it would be useful in the early screening of appropriate job openings. A request for typical information relevant to one person may be made when the characteristics of that person are known.

Another brief analysis form is illustrated in Table 2. This form permits the analyzer to quickly consider a person's capabilities and limitations with respect to job characteristics. Such a form can indicate what particular job/person areas need more in-depth study. A careful preview analysis can help an analyzer decide how to allocate time and thus make job analyses more efficient. This analysis form also indicates areas in which environmental modifications might be appropriate. This signals areas in which a person with a disability might consider personal adaptations where environmental changes may be too costly or difficult. Thus, this type of preliminary analysis can be useful to plan for additional rehabilitation services.

If occupational adjustment is to continue to be significant in rehabilitation planning, individuals and their counselors must have accurate and adequate job information so that they can make educated decisions about what changes must be made. For instance if a job requires that one work rapidly for long periods, that one have a strong back and hands, that foot-hand-eye coordination is important, or that one must be able to estimate size and speed of objects, then the job-seeker had better know this before taking the job. Thus, this information is essential to anyone who provides services that help people prepare for work.

Other uses of job analysis include:

1. Job analysis provides occupational data so that employee performance on the job can be evaluated. Worker qualifications and abilities can then be related to requirements and demands so that employee performance requirements can be objectively determined.
2. A successful training program depends in part upon detailed information regarding jobs. Workers cannot be trained adequately unless such matters as the nature, duties, and responsibilities of the jobs for which they are being trained are known.
3. Safety engineers take job analysis into account to locate potential occupational hazards and to develop safety procedures that will eliminate hazards.

Table 1.   Abbreviated job analysis form

1. Company name _____ Date _____	
2. Personnel manager's name _____ Title _____	
3. Company address _____ Telephone no. _____	
4. Types of jobs (entry level and other) _____	
5. Salaries (entry level and other) _____	
6. Number of shifts and hours _____ Union? _____	
7. How and/or where do they find their employees? _____	
8. What is their selection procedure? Tastes?_____	
9. Do they currently have any handicapped workers? What has been their experience? _____	
10. Have they been contacted by Vocational Rehabilitation, Goodwill, or other agencies? Explain _____	
11. What is their (real) attitude about hiring the handicapped? _____	
12. Further comments about the company, personnel manager, location for transportation, etc. _____	
13. Personal reactions and comments_____	

From Engelkes (1968) by permission.

Table 2.   Critical items analysis

Job:

Job duties:

		Physical demands		
Client	Activity	Percent of time	Weight/Distance	Accommodations
	Walking			
	Standing			
	Seeing			
	Hearing			
		Work environment		
Client	Obstacles	Adaptations		
	Door			
	Desk			
	Toilet			
	Cafeteria			
	Parking			

From Human Resources Center (1978) by permission.

4. Job descriptions obtained from the job analysis are also valuable means of identifying jobs that are closely allied. This information can prove helpful in moving workers from job to job within the same plant or in the same community (Office of the Governor of Texas, 1975).

5. A series of analysis of jobs that exist in an organization can identify the skills and experiences needed to advance through these jobs. In this way, counselors can help people plan for career development while they are still in the rehabilitation process.

SPECIAL CONSIDERATIONS FOR JOB ANALYSIS CONCERNING PERSONS WITH VARIOUS DISABILITIES

A person with a disability involving mobility limitations needs a particularly detailed analysis of both the work and home environment. It is likely for such a person to need assistance in analyzing the home for self-care; such things as dressing, bathing, hygiene, eating, hand manipulation, pinch, grasp, coordination, and endurance must all be considered.

Evaluation of the environment should by nature include making note of techniques of physical transfer around home, transportation, transfers necessary at work, communication, architectural barriers, and other necessary adaptations to facilitate moving between home and work. Evaluation should also be concerned with work tolerance, work productivity, attitudes of co-workers and supervisors, and the informal social context within which one lives and works. Motivation, judgment, reading comprehension, mathematical aptitude, vocational potential, and general emotional adjustment should also be evaluated to assure the rehabilitation professional that all the significant variables associated with work placement and adjustment have been covered.

The mentally retarded require special consideration on the part of the rehabilitation professional conducting job analysis. Special attention must be paid to the complexity of the job itself. Frequently, jobs being performed need only consist of several simple tasks: the analysis must determine whether a few complex tasks have been included to add some enrichment to the job. Hiring requirements suggesting that one have a high school diploma could be invalid except for the complex tasks assigned to that job. Perhaps the tasks may be broken down or recombined so that new, simpler jobs could be created that would facilitate the hiring of retarded people. At the same time, careful assessment of the retarded person's capabilities should be made. It is possible that retarded workers will be able to perform well enough physically or mentally so that they can complete circumscribed sets of complex tasks. Whenever possible, retarded individuals should be encouraged to obtain employment that they can perform and that will also be personally and socially satisfying.

Special considerations need to be made for conducting job analysis with the emotionally disturbed person in mind, too. *Emotionally disturbed* is a term that lumps a variety of psychopathological entities together, yet obviously not all emotionally disturbed individuals are the same. Careful assessment of the problems of these individuals should be made. The difficulties they are experiencing should be understood and their strengths should be matched to jobs that will capitalize on them. In cases in which the job-seeker is emotionally disturbed, the counselor conducting a job analysis should pay special attention to the general job environment, the variety or routine of tasks to be performed, the nature of the supervision to be given, the nature of the relationships with co-workers within that department or unit, and the nature and amount of psychological support available at home, from the rehabilitation or psychological professional, or from friends.

All of the special considerations reported here must be taken into account to assure appropriate placement. Several of these considerations suggest job restructuring. This chapter would not be complete without at least some reference to this concept and its relationship to job analysis.

RELATIONSHIP OF JOB ANALYSIS TO JOB RESTRUCTURING

Job restructuring is a special application of job analysis that involves viewing jobs within the context of the system of which they are a part, analyzing them, and then rearranging their tasks to achieve a desired end (United States Department of Labor, 1970). Although the term *job restructuring* is relatively new, the concept is not. At times, employers find it necessary to rearrange or to adjust the contents (tasks performed) of jobs within a system. This can happen when economic conditions change, when technological advances are made, if vacant positions cannot be filled, or if federal regulations governing employment practices are revised. Job restructuring may also be considered by employers so that rehabilitated workers can be hired.

A job does not exist alone but is related to a number of other jobs in a system in which interdependencies and relationships among the jobs cannot be ignored. Job restructuring should be thought of not as changing one job, but rather as rearranging the contents of jobs within a system.

Job analysis is the basic technique used in job restructuring. Any activity in this area should begin with identification of the jobs within a system and analysis of the separate tasks that comprise each of the jobs, followed by evaluation of the characteristics and relationships of the tasks involved. Each job must be analyzed in terms of:

1. The specific tasks performed by the worker
2. The functioning of the worker in relation to data, people, and things
3. The minimum general educational development required for satisfactory performance
4. An estimation of the aptitudes required for satisfactory job performance by the worker
5. Other significant worker trait requirements, such as physical demands, temperaments, and interests

The methodology of restructuring is an outgrowth of the widely held belief that better utilization of the available labor force can alleviate many labor problems. The potential of the labor force for complex work can be developed through on-the-job training and experience. Major goals of training programs are, first, to increase employment opportunities at the entry level for persons who do not possess the necessary skills to compete in the labor market and, second, to create meaningful opportunities so that these people will advance to higher level jobs as they acquire new skills. One way to achieve these goals is through application of job restructuring techniques.

Job restructuring yields some immediate benefits. It frees experienced personnel to spend more time performing higher level tasks and creates lower level jobs that can be filled by inexperienced persons. A significant result of this is new employment opportunites, not only for persons with disabilities but also for youth entering the labor market for the first time or for those re-entering the labor market after a hiatus taken, for example, to raise a family.

More efficient utilization of labor force resources will result in higher labor productivity. In job restructuring, the analyst should be interested not only in creating entry-level positions, but also in trying to devise meaningful promotional opportunities. The job restructuring methodology enables the analyst to design a series of career lattices. The career lattice uses the interrelationships among jobs to create promotional opportunities and facilitate mobility for workers among jobs. This mobility is provided by a career lattice in three directions—horizontal mobility to jobs at the same relative level of complexity but in different areas of work, vertical mobility to more complex jobs in the same areas of work, and diagonal mobility to more complex jobs in a different but related area of work (Norris et al., 1979). In this way, rehabilitation professionals can help people with disabilities achieve a better measure of career development.

SUMMARY

Every rehabilitation professional uses job analysis information, whether it is referred to as such or not. When systematic job analyses are made, the counselor has better organized and more extensive knowledge about 1) business and industry in general and 2) the specifiç jobs represented by those businesses and industries in particular. The rehabilitation professional's increased knowledge serves as a useful aid to persons with disabilities and employers in differential job selection or placement. A job analysis is simply an organized way of learning about the important aspects of a job. In placement, it provides a useful, organized system of job-relevant knowledge that can be of aid to a person who is seeking help in the placement process.

Special attention must be paid to job duties for the sake of persons who have certain disabilities. The mobility-impaired individual needs special focus on the mobility improvement potential. When working with mentally retarded persons, the complexity of a job deserves extra attention. Emotionally disturbed persons need special support systems for themselves at work or at home.

Finally, job restructuring is related to job analysis. This is one area in which rehabilitation professionals can increase their value to employers as they help them prepare lattices for career development.

REFERENCES

Bowman, J. T., and Graves, W. H. 1976. Placement Services and Techniques. Stipes Publishing Co., Champaign, Illinois.

Engelkes, J. R. 1968. Occupational information. *In* L. A. Miller and C. E. Oberman (eds.), Studies in the Continuing Education of Rehabilitation Counselors. University of Iowa, Iowa City.

Engelkes, J. R. 1978. Job analysis in vocational rehabilitation. Prepared for University of Nebraska—Lincoln National Short-term Training, Project sponsored by Rehabilitation Services Administration on job analysis, job modification, and job forecasting.

Human Resources Center. 1978. Module 12: Job analysis. *In* Modular Placement Training Package. Author. Albertson, New York.

Mallik, K., and Sablowsky, R. 1975. Model for placement: Job laboratory approach. J. Rehab. 41:14–20, 41.

Nadler, G. 1963. Work Designs. Irwin Publishers, Chicago.

Norris, W., Hatch, R. N., Engelkes, J. R., and Winborn, B. B. 1979. The Career Information Service. Rand McNally & Co., Chicago.

Office of the Governor of Texas. 1975. Participants handbook, governmental supervisors training program. Texas Rehabilitation Commission, Austin.

United States Department of Labor, Manpower Administration. 1970. Handbook for Job Restructuring. Author. Washington, D.C.

United States Department of Labor, Manpower Administration. 1972. Handbook for Analyzing Jobs. Author. Washington, D.C.

Chapter 8

Job Accommodation through Job Restructuring and Environmental Modification

Kalisankar Mallik

Editor's note: This chapter can be regarded as a sequel to the previous chapter, since the functions of job restructuring and environmental modification depend on information obtained from job analysis. The author illustrates the value job analysis can have within the total rehabilitation process. Even in this area, however, approaches can differ. The previous chapter suggests how job analysis might be useful for specific clients who need specific types of jobs. This chapter on accommodations cautions that the job analyzer must be careful not to let concern for the placement of a particular client interfere with an objective job analysis. This point does not negate the use of job analysis for planning individual rehabilitation, but it places appropriate emphasis on the need for objectivity.

This chapter also illustrates how rehabilitation can benefit from the expertise of bioengineering. The technology available from this science has direct use in the placement of people with disabilities, particularly for those with severe functional limitations. The Job Development Laboratory has demonstrated that persons believed to be unplaceable have achieved competitive employment and maintained production requirements through appropriate job restructuring and environmental modification.

Of course, not every counselor can have a bioengineer as a ready resource. This chapter recognizes this problem and emphasizes that many accommodations result from a new way of analyzing a situation when one realizes that many adaptations are simple and often require only the creativity to recognize that a common item, cheaply available, can be used to open a whole new area of functioning for a person with a disability. Often, after a situation has been carefully analyzed, a counselor and client might together develop an accommodation. This process can also be a valuable learning experience for the client, useful over a lifetime. The client has probably developed many adaptations and a systematic approach could provide much success. This chapter also aids the counselor by cataloging, in one document, many commercial devices relevant for overcoming a variety of functional limitations. A list of manufacturers, as well as references, is provided to enable the interested person to make further inquiry.

JOB RESTRUCTURING OR JOB TASK MODIFICATION

Job restructuring is a process through which one combines, eliminates, redistributes, adds, or isolates tasks from one or more jobs within the same job family to form part-time or full-time positions. Possible advantages of restructuring include a better use of the available work force, enhancement of overall performance, assistance in developing job opportunities, and facilitation of upward mobility. Possible disadvantages include the need for psychological adjustment, an increase in skill specialization, and adjustment to new tasks.

Before modifying or reengineering a job, one should know what relevant tasks are associated with the job or position (a particular defined job within a section is called a *position*), and who is going to perform the job tasks. This knowledge can best be ascertained through a job/position task analysis, an individual functional analysis, and a job-client matching process.

The key point to remember in job analysis is that the job tasks have to be performed effectively. A job analysis cannot be done properly if the analyst comes to work with a bias, such as an a priori desire to place a particular person in a job. The job should be analyzed objectively according to its own physical and cognitive requirements. This is the only way a potential employer can come to feel that serious business interests are not being overlooked and that a cooperative relationship is being established between the counselor and employer. A good working relationship is particularly essential when developing homebound positions, since doing so often depends on the rehabilitation professional's ability to make the advantages of hiring these workers clear.

It is common practice for large organizations to require all employees in a particular work section consisting of 20 to 30 employees to be able to perform each and every task related to the work flow of that section. Usually, some of the work in such an office can be done at home. For instance, the job tasks that must be performed in one "order processing section" of a large organization include: bringing the mail from the mailroom, sorting and stapling it, stamping it with the date and time, and logging the mail in. Next, a process begins that involves coding and entering information into a computer, retrieving information, delivering relevant documents to appropriate sections, and so on. While the mail-handling operations would certainly be inappropriate for consideration as a homebound job, the computer entry and retrieval operations might well be done effectively by a homebound employee using a remote computer terminal. If all employees are required to do all operations within this section, homebound employment is impossible. However, if the work flow is task reorganized so that a limited number of employees are responsible for certain tasks, a homebound employee can be added to the staff.

Usually, employers expect all workers to perform all tasks in a work section so that attrition will not disrupt the job flow of the section. This precaution need not be sacrificed by reorganizing to accommodate a homebound employee. The employer can avoid work loss by dividing the total number of tasks into four or five subgroups and periodically rotating the duties of the on-site employees.

Reorganizing the methods and techniques of distributing tasks in an office to accommodate a particular homebound or on-site employee can be achieved without lowering productivity if employers and rehabilitation professionals work together. The positive results of such cooperation have already been shown by employers working with the staff of the Job Development Laboratory at George Washington University. Many persons with severe disabilities have become productive homebound and on-site employees of such organizations as the Insurance Company of North America, Rehab Group, Inc., Info-Con, Inc., General Services Administration, Office of Human Development, Social Rehabilitation Services Administration, United States Customs, Department of Justice, and the Food and Drug Administration. Supervisors from these organizations have cooperated in restructuring or reorganizing the job tasks of their departments, opening new doors for people with disabilities. This job restructuring (or job task modification) technique aids in job-client matching, which ultimately minimizes the costs of environmental modifications through assistive devices, engineering approaches, or training.

ENVIRONMENTAL MODIFICATION

Environmental modification is a process that provides aids for people or alters their physical or attitudinal surroundings. Such modifications may produce many advantages, which contribute to the maximization of the effectiveness of human resources. These advantages include improvements in productivity, versatility and adaptability on the part of the worker; an increased capacity to perform wider ranges of tasks; and a reduction of fatigue resulting from job tasks. Furthermore, environmental modifications can lead to the simplification of perceptual, physical, and cognitive tasks, which can reduce the time and motion required for job tasks.

It is important to recognize, however, that there are potential disadvantages to pursuing environmental modifications. Some of these are increased costs to the business involved, a danger of oversimplifying job tasks, which would make job routines monotonous, and a complication of maintenance procedures.

Environmental modifications are expected to increase opportunities for participation in the labor market for persons with severe disabilities. People whose functional limitations are severe face potential vocational barriers in environments in which they live. These barriers can be minimized through judicious modification. The question of modifying employer and co-worker attitudes toward persons with disabilities has received a good deal of attention in other publications, and therefore is not addressed in this chapter. Rather, the general intention here is to discuss various methods by which people with severe disabilities can be competitively employed at home or at on-site jobs. Specific attention is paid to the use of low-cost, simple adaptations that enhance independent work functioning in the areas of gaining access to source documents, improving communications, using equipment, increasing mobility, and other activities of daily living. Improving architectural accessibility for people with disabilities is also discussed. A brief description of various devices designed and constructed at the Job Development Laboratory is included in this chapter. Where appropriate, various devices are discussed with relation to specific disabilities. Many adaptive devices are now commercially available. Some sources for obtaining such devices are named in the discussion that follows to show how the reader can find imaginative and creative solutions to functional problems through the use of low-cost, simple adaptations.

Gaining Access to Source Documents

Many people who are victims of accident or disease have limitations in reach, are confined to wheelchairs, and must overcome man-made obstacles everyday. In an office, such a person faces difficulties in using the surface of a desk, moving about within a building, and reaching files that are kept at various heights. The problem is more severe if individuals have limited or no use of their hands, arms and shoulder muscles, or paralysis of all extremities. Because individuals in these disability groups are most likely to need desk jobs, the ability to reach source documents is crucial to their vocational success (Mallik, 1975; Mallik and Sablowsky, 1975). Such source documents as the telephone directory, books explaining how to code information, office files, forms, reference books, reports, journal articles, and invoices are essential to office work. If necessary, suitable modifications should be made so that an individual can reach the documents easily, even with limited functional capabilities (Mallik and Mueller, 1975, 1977).

Modifications in the environment may include placement of file stacks at appropriate height and reach or reducing the height of file cabinets with easy-opening cabinet door mechanisms. Documents can be microfilmed to provide access to information and at the same time eliminate the strength and precise manipulation required for lifting documents and turning pages. Information can be programmed into a personal terminal from a remote computer and retrieved by using keyboards. An adjustable table/desk can be provided so that individuals can reach the desk surface without fatiguing hand and shoulder muscles.

A simple aid for people with limited reach or grasp is an "automatic page turner," which holds books or magazines at the proper reading angle and turns pages with the slightest touch (Mallik and Mueller, 1977; HB & D Products; Touch Turner Company). Devices are available that turn one page at a time, either forward or backward. Once a book is slipped inside the device and the proper angle is adjusted, reading is feasible in bed, in a wheelchair, or at a table. A portable page turner with a rechargeable battery is also available.

Another device is the "Ealing Reader," in which a continuous clear plastic sleeve (150 feet long with 150 pockets to contain as many pages) is rolled onto a spool, and is snapped into place in a cassette (The Ealing Corporation). The sleeve is threaded through the cassette and attached to a take-up spool. Two copies of the reading material (e.g., textbook, journal) are taken apart and inserted in the pockets of the plastic sleeve. (Two copies are required because the pages cannot be turned over to read the reverse side.) The cassette is placed inside the device, which rolls the tape forward and back when a switch that requires only a few ounces of force is activated.

Visually impaired people who have no other physical limitations can get information through optical aids ("Optical Aids Service—Survey," 1957). Examples of such aids are hand magnifying glasses with or without illumination ("Low Vision Service," 1974), reading machines (Visualtek, "What a Visualtek Can Do") or raised letters on file cabinets.

A device called the Optacon has been used effectively to solve the source document access problems of totally blind people, provided they do not have any loss of tactile stimulation of their fingers (Telesensory Systems, Inc.). The Pew Memorial Trust of Philadelphia is making it possible for the Volunteer Services for the Blind to train Optacon users and provide Optacons to them at reduced cost.

For educable, mentally retarded people, access to documents can be improved through the use of various search techniques, which can be alphabetical, numerical, chronological, or can involve special symbols. However, trainable mentally retarded persons at lower levels may have difficulties understanding documents. In this case, easily comprehensible sequencing techniques are recommended.

Communication

The telephone is one of the basic tools through which a person can maintain communication with the community and particularly with fellow workers and supervisors (Sullivan, Frieden, and Cordery, 1968). Simple tasks, such as lifting and holding a telephone receiver while dialing, can present a problem for the person with minimal grasp, elbow extension and flexion, and finger strength. A flexible extension (goose neck) attached to a Touch-Tone phone, which holds the receiver for the person, or a headphone set with a Touch-Tone phone can solve these problems. Communication control systems have been available for people who have no use of hand, arm, and shoulder muscles (BARD/CARBA Division; Down East Electronics Manufacturing Company; Fidelity Electronics, Ltd.). These systems give persons with disabilities unaided access to a telephone, control of a television or radio, control of room lights, and a variety of other functions. Functions can be selected by a tongue control switch or a puff/sip (breath control) on a plastic tube attached to the control.

A person with deafness may face no problem in communicating with others through use of a teletypewriter (TTY). With this device, messages are typewritten rather than audible.

Other communication aids that have been designed for the deaf include:

1. A battery-operated "Light Writer" developed by Churchill, of England. This consists of a 32-character electronic display. The display is removable so it can be placed at a desired position.
2. The "MCM" (Manual Communication Module), a portable electronic device designed for telephone or vocal communication by Micon Industries, Oakland, California. This device is used by the deaf, hearing impaired, nonverbal individuals and their families.
3. The "Talking Brooch" is a portable device primarily for mute individuals designed by the University of Southhampton, England. This battery-powered aid has a five-character display, which fits on the shirt pocket like a brooch with a separate keyboard (Vanderheiden and Grilley, 1975).

Writing is another method of communication that should not be overlooked. If the individual is not able to write due to impaired hand function, then alternative approaches must be explored. Among the methods used by the Job Development Laboratory is "tenodesis." This device is a hand orthotic device which transfers the function of wrist flexion and extension to the fingers to facilitate pinch and grasp. So equipped, an individual can utilize electric typewriters (with or without a hand rest or keyboard guard), adapted tape recorders (which can be used as notebooks), and rubber stamps (which are useful if words need to be printed repeatedly).

Persons who cannot use handwriting as a mode of communication frequently use a typewriter. Those who have spastic or athetoid cerebral palsy, however, cannot exercise precise control over the movements of their fingers. As a result, they make typing errors. To help those suffering from such severe motor problems, electric typewriters can be equipped with enlarged keyboards, which can be fitted to some commercially available models (BARD/CARBA, PMV system). There are many other communication aids, devices, and systems available for persons with severe disabilities. A good deal of helpful information can be found in a book entitled *Communication for the Developmentally Disabled: A Resource Guide for Parents and Professionals* (Mallik et al., 1977).

Many other communication devices and systems have already been developed through research and demonstration efforts (Kafafian, 1970, 1973; Nickerson and Stevens, 1976; National Institute for Rehab. Engineering, 1973). If they were made available nationally, they would enhance the communication efforts of many persons with severe disabilities.

UTILIZATION OF OFFICE AND HOME EQUIPMENT DEVICES

Many jobs require equipment operation in order to accomplish one or more tasks (Leslie et al., 1976; Mallik and Shworles, 1971; Shworles and Mallik, 1971a, b). Usually, performance features and control switches on such equipment are not designed for an operator with a disability ("The Handicapped Majority," 1974). Small knobs, for example, are often difficult for an impaired hand to squeeze or turn. If this is the case, a small knob can be replaced by a larger knob or lever whose manipulation requires less than usual strength and dexterity. All switches should be modified so that they can be activated with only a few ounces of force. They should also be placed in positions that minimize fatigue and enhance productivity.

A pneumatic holding device, for example, can grasp and release a piece that is otherwise difficult for a cerebral palsied individual to hold while operating a drill press. "Hold" and "release" modes are activated by a microswitch, which is placed at the best location for the worker. There are various types of controllers available. A few of them are as follows:

1. Chin control (can be worn or fixed in the desired location)
2. Head control (left/right or forward/backward movement)
3. Joystick control (electric wheelchairs use this type of control)
4. Tongue control (activated by tongue movement)
5. Shoulder control (elevation and depression of shoulder)
6. Pneumatic control (puff/sip)
7. Eyelid control (microswitch is mounted on spectacles)
8. Voice control (unit is trained on individual's voice frequency)
9. Ultrasonic control (operates remotely by a sound)
10. Radio control (similar to garage door opener)

The Environmental Control unit initially designed by the VAPC (Veterans Administration Prosthetics Center) is now available commercially (General Teleoperators, Inc.). This device permits completely immobilized individuals to operate or control common electrical appliances located in the hospital, home, or office. Wheelchair-based environmental control is also feasible (Romich, Beery and Bayer, Inc.). This sort of device operates the electric wheelchair, a powered splint (orthotic device), lap-board-mounted tape recorder, powered recliner, radio, respirator, door openers, or other equipment. Other environmental control units that can operate these appliances, along with typewriters and page turners, are indicated in sections "Gaining Access to Source Documents" and "Communication."

The "Speech and Talking Calculator," a hand-held or tabletop electronic calculator, is now available commercially (American Foundation for the Blind, Telesensory Systems, Inc.). Blind individuals may find it useful at home, in the classroom, and at work. Also, technological advancement has made it possible to command a computer using a voice input terminal (Scope Electronics, Inc.). People who have no hand function or head rotation are now being trained as computer programmers and data entry operators using this system. The training is organized by the Job Development Laboratory of George Washington University.

The creation of a computer that can "speak" is of great concern to many organizations for the blind. Massachusetts Institute of Technology of Boston and Telsensory Systems, Inc., of Palo Alto have made tremendous progress in determining the feasibility of a direct translation/speech output reading system ("TSI's Computer Now Reads," TSI Newsletter #15).

Deaf persons may find it hard to use some types of equipment. For example, a microfilm camera indicates by sound that the film unit is out of film or that the film unit is not placed properly. Barriers for employment can be eliminated using other signals, such as light indicators or vibrations.

Multiply impaired and mentally retarded persons may confront a variety of environmental barriers which, although discouraging, can be rather easily overcome. The use of a record player can be simplified by using cast polyester control knobs. Address labels can be more easily applied using a labeling guide. These guides are particularly helpful in a sheltered work situation. Also important for workshop production are magnetically adjusted paper folding guides. Paper money dispensers can be useful both at work and privately. All of these modifications have implications for improving the quality of work, as well as improving life in general.

People with spasticity or athetosis may still be capable of operating equipment if their hands can be stabilized on a platform while they work. For the severely cerebral palsied person, stabilization of the entire body is usually necessary. The lower part of the body can be stabilized by anchoring the crossed legs to one leg of the wheelchair. The upper part of the body can be anchored by the nondominant hand if necessary. There are still other techniques of positioning, a few of which are indicated in the section on mobility.

MOBILITY

Problems in mobility for persons with severe disabilities vary greatly according to the type of mobility required (Brown, 1975). The mobility levels can be classified broadly into the following categories:

1. Mobility in the home or at a work site
2. Mobility within the neighborhood or community
3. Mobility from one community to another community
4. Mobility from one city to another

Items 1 and 2 may not be a problem to those with less severe disabilities, but they may present serious problems to those who have more severe functional limitations. Persons confined to a manual wheelchair may become tired from the act of maneuvering the wheelchair. Deep pile carpeting may make the use of crutches and walkers difficult. The solution to this problem is to cover rugs with plastic mats or get rid of carpeting altogether. Another common problem is that of doorway access and doorknob manipulation. Solutions to these problems may be found in widening the doorways, reducing the tension of the door, installing an electric door opening/closing mechanism, or replacing doorknobs with levers (Jamero, 1976; Kliment, 1975).

If stair climbing is a problem, then a home elevator may be a solution (Earl's Stairway Lift Corporation). This lift can be installed in closet space, stairwells, corners, or the side of a room. For accommodating 3' × 4' lift, a 3'9" × 4'3" clear space is recommended. Another solution for stair climbing is a "stair-climbing elevator" or "stair glider" (The Cheney Company; Earl's Stairway Lift Corporation). This is an electrically driven chair that glides on a rail that is installed on one side of a staircase.

Frequently, a few steps in front of a house or a building pose an architectural barrier for a person using a walker, crutches, or a wheelchair. The solution to this problem may be a ramp or a wheelchair lift (American Manufacturing Company, Inc.; Handi-Ramp, Inc.; Toce Brothers Manufacturing Ltd.).

A person confined to a wheelchair finds it particularly difficult to move from place to place. Proper selection of the wheelchair not only aids in comfort but also helps to increase mobility. Everest and Jennings, Inc., in one of its publications, "Modification and Accessory Analysis," suggests that the advantages and limitations of various parts of a wheelchair need to be considered before a person selects one. The following is an example (taken from the aforementioned document):

A. 5" Diameter Casters (front wheels)

Advantages	*Limitations*
Lighter than 8" casters	Should be used on smooth surfaces
	Difficult to operate over obstructions, such as rug edges, thresholds, and rough sidewalks
	Not recommended for lawns or rough ground

B. 8" Diameter Casters

Advantages	*Limitations*
Rolls easily over rough ground	Slightly heavier than 5" diameter casters
Swivels easily	
Helps to absorb road shock	
Double ball bearing in stem gives longer life	
Interchangeable with semi-pneumatic tires	
Caster swivel locks may be used	

Similarly, the document covers the advantages and limitations of other items, such as:

1. Chair size (adult, narrow adult, junior-16, junior-13, growing chair, tiny-tot high, tiny-tot low)
2. Arm type (fixed, detachable, adjustable, rotating, armless)
3. Frame construction (light, heavy, indoor, outdoor)
4. Back style (upright, semi-reclining, full reclining, zipper back, safety belt)
5. Foot and leg support (swinging, detachable, permanent, adjustable, ankle strap, toe strap, heel strap)

6. Drive (manual, power drive—proportional or microswitch)
7. Wheels (pneumatic, semi-pneumatic, handrims, handrims—plastic coated)

These items indicate that a wheelchair cannot merely be defined as a chair with wheels. The acquisition of a wheelchair is based on consideration of both the availability of various kinds of wheelchairs on the market and the individual's need and preference (American Stair-Glide Corporation; Invacare Corporation; Institutional Industries; J. A. Preston Corporation; Lakeside Manufacturing Inc.). The individual's need is based on the nature of the impairment, an analysis of how greatly movement is limited, and such problems as susceptibility of skin to breakdown, limited balance, bed sores, or other pain.

Blind people encounter special kinds of mobility problems, although mobility is not always difficult and most often people who are blind can manage with a long cane or a guide dog. The Sonic-Guide, an electronic mobility aid and environmental sensor, can enhance and extend the independent travel of blind individuals (Telesensory Systems, Inc.). A small transmitter located in a lightweight spectacle frame radiates ultrasound (high frequency sound inaudible to the human ear) in front of the wearer. When the ultrasound hits an object, such as a wall or a tree, it is reflected back to the aid. The ultrasound is then converted into audible sound, which is diverted into the ears by small ear tubes. This device is generally used in conjunction with a long cane or a guide dog.

Long-range mobility, such as levels 3 and 4, depend on the availability of accessible transportation systems. A cab may be used by many people who have manual wheelchairs. Electric wheelchairs, however, pose many problems, one of which is the transport of the chair. For this reason, persons requiring the use of electric wheelchairs should, if possible, purchase a specialized van that is equipped with a manual, hydraulic, or electric ramp or lift (Double Industries, Inc.; Para Industries, Ltd.; Telesensory Systems, Inc.). Persons with various kinds of impairments can drive a van or regular car using proper hand controls and hand orthotic devices to stabilize the forearm and hand. These devices also increase strength needed to operate the steering wheel and lever for acceleration and brakes (Gresham Driving Aids, Inc., "You Too, Can Drive!"). Many persons confined to a manual wheelchair who can drive cars using hand controls may find it difficult to load and unload their wheelchairs. The "Mark VII Loader" was designed to solve this problem. This electromechanical device can be installed on the top of the car and it receives electrical power from the 12-volt car battery (The Wheelchair Carrier Corporation). This device allows the person to remove or replace the wheelchair without any assistance. Another helpful device called "Lowry" is now in production (Innovations, Inc.). People with scoliosis or osteogenesis may find it difficult to maintain a regular sitting posture and stability. Several persons with these impairments, having availed themselves of the services of the Job Development Laboratory, are now driving their automobiles with the help of contour seats and leg supports.

Other devices that have been used to facilitate longer range travel include overwheel transfer boards for the person with limited use of shoulder and hand muscles. These transfer boards help stabilize the transfer of the person from the wheelchair to a car or vice versa. Another device is a helmet cover for epileptic persons who may have seizures without warning. These people may face a health problem in mobility as a result of falling. If the individual prefers not to wear an unattractive protective helmet, an alternative is using a wheelchair, which would eliminate the problem of falling but would create other special problems in mobility. A more suitable solution, however, may be covering the helmet with a turban or a wig, making it less noticeable and more attractive.

Inter-city mobility not only depends on local transportation, but also on the accessibility of trains, buses, planes, and their respective terminals (Thomas Built Buses, Inc.; Viking, "Van Tops"; Annand, 1971; National Railroad Passenger Corporation, 1977). Extensive checking and planning is necessary when long-range travel is attempted.

For the homebound employee the question may arise: Why should mobility anywhere besides home be important? The answer is that many of the jobs that persons with severe disabilities can do require specialized community-based training or on-the-job training before a homebound job begins. Sometimes homebound individuals must visit their employers once a week or once a month for work assignments, special discussions, further training, or to discuss a decision-making process.

The Job Development Laboratory at George Washington University finds this interaction between homebound persons and their supervisors constructive and stimulating. Under the circumstances, the homebound person does not feel totally isolated from society, and through this interaction many who have used the Job Development Laboratory become non-homebound once they acquire economic independence.

ACTIVITIES OF DAILY LIVING

Activities of Daily Living (ADL) include training in various self-care tasks, such as dressing, bathing, oral hygiene, eating, manipulation, mobility, and communication. If a person spends a considerable amount of time and energy doing these activities, then a limited amount of energy will be left for vocational pursuits. Such an uneven expenditure of energy deprives an individual of the chance to be a productive worker, whether homebound or employed away from home. An evaluation of self-care activities assists the rehabilitation professional in determining the client's ability to adapt, compensate for, or perform job tasks optimally.

When considering ADL, comfort becomes an important concern. Persons confined to wheelchairs may find sitting for a long time on any wheelchair cushion uncomfortable. There are however, many types of commercial wheelchair cushions available, and one may help. A few of them are as follows:

1. Checker board T-Foam Cushions (Alimed). This laminated duplex cushion consists of two layers:
    a. an upper layer of cubes (250 individual cubes arranged like a checkerboard), high density foam
    b. a self-contouring T-Foam base. The inherent moldability of the T-Foam base gives the fluid/foam feeling familiar to T-Foam users. The cushion is covered with knit polyester for maximum breathability, ease of transfer, and optimum pressure distribution. The forward (leg edge) of checkerboard cushions is tapered to maximize transition pressure at the cushion termination under the thigh.
2. T-Foam Cushion.
3. "Mud" Cushion.
4. "Gel" Pad (Bio Clinic Company).
5. "Flotation" Pad (Bio Clinic Company).
6. "ROHO" dry flotation pad (Accurate Medical Service).

Persons susceptible to pressure sores may have a problem using mattresses. This is particularly true when the person cannot turn over without physical assistance. The Frusto-Conical Mattress or Ripple Bed (size 2'10" × 5'6", weight 11 pounds) consists of a base sheet membrane, air cells (14 cells along the width of the mattress), twin bore air supply manifold, and an optional protective cover (Tally Surgical Instruments, Ltd.). This ripple bed is operated by a power unit, which has a provision for controlling a chair-cushion. The power unit generates cycles every 10 minutes.

Many high-level spinal cord injured persons who have little or no control of their bladders generally use an external urinary catheter. The external male urinary catheter consists of a lightweight latex sheath, securely attached to a universal connector and accompanied by a high quality elastic foam strap (Intermed Associates, Inc.). This is used on males to direct the flow of urine into a suitable receptacle called a urinary leg bag. External female urinary catheters are available, but these require diligent attention to prevent rashes and other skin reactions. Most females use internal catherization.

Emptying urinary leg bags is a problem for the nurse, attendant, or client. A leg bag valve mechanism is the Leg Urinal Drain Valve (EZMT Valve Company), a valve that operates with only one finger. When released, the valve closes automatically. This lightweight drain valve can be installed to any standard leg bag. Also, the Clip-Drain (Intermed Associates, Inc.), a one-piece molded light weight plastic clamp valve with $\frac{9}{32}$" latex tubing, 5" in length, is available. It is attached to the bottom of the urinary leg bag to facilitate emptying. Complete shutoff is accomplished with a control ratchet operated with one hand and opened with the thumb.

Persons confined to a wheelchair who have impaired upper extremities always find difficulties in the transfer process. The transfer may be from wheelchair to bed, to car, to bathtub, to swimming pool, to commode, or vice versa. Hoyer lifters can assist such transfers with minimum assistance (Ted Hoyer & Company, Inc.). This hydraulic or mechanical jack, which rotates 180°, has a locking device at the lower end of the mast, which locks the mast and base together. This allows the user to have the option of locking the mast and base together or unlocking the mast from the base for transport or storage.

There are many other commercially available devices that can assist handicapped people to be self-sufficient in activities of daily living (G. E. Miller, Inc., Catalog 95; Hausman Industries, Inc., "Equipment for Health Care and Rehabilitation"; J. A. Preston Corporation, Catalog 1095; Lumex, Inc., "Patient Aids"; Medical Equipment Distributors, Catalogs 1a and 2; Triaxon, Inc. (Aqualift); McCluer et al., 1974; Melichar, 1974; Product/Service Buyer's Guide for the Rehabilitation Industries, 1976). Sometimes it is necessary to provide a minor modification or adjustment to these devices according to the individual's need. Generally, modifications can be made by an occupational therapist, a physical therapist, an engineer, a designer, or even by a family member. There are many cases, however, in which a person's limitations are so severe or so specialized that the existing devices are inadequate to ensure independence. In those cases, some imagination on the part of people with experience in rehabilitation must be brought to bear on the problem (Lowman and Klinger, 1969; Robinault, 1973; Macey, 1974; Howard, 1975; Mallik and Yuspeh, 1975). The opinions and suggestions of the individual who requires such special help are vital in helping to resolve a particular difficulty.

Sometimes solutions involve extraordinarily simple modifications. The Job Development Laboratory staff used some ingenuity and a low-cost, simple adaptation to increase independence for a disabled woman in this way: D. L. was offered a position in data entry operations at the U.S. Civil Service Commission. Although the rest room was accessible to her wheelchair, she had insufficient strength and stamina to transfer to the commode. Commercial transfer aids were inadequate and hand-held urine containers were inappropriate for the sitting position. After exploration of available containers, a laundry detergent bottle was modified for easy use and emptying from the sitting position. Total cost of the device (including detergent) was $1.59.

ARCHITECTURAL ACCESSIBILITY

Stephen A. Kliment of the Department of Health, Education and Welfare made the following remarks in his booklet "Into the Mainstream—A Syllabus for a Barrier Free Environment" (1975):

> In the United States today, it is estimated that one out of ten persons has limited mobility due to a temporary or a permanent physical handicap. This number may be increasing due to improved medical techniques which provide some mobility where it was not possible in the past. Also the expanding population of older persons contributes additional numbers. Yet in general, the physical environment of our nation's communities continues to be designed to accommodate the ablebodied, thereby perpetuating the isolation and dependence of disabled persons. To break this pattern requires a national commitment.

Rules and regulations have been set up to eliminate architectural barriers. Most federal buildings or federally funded facilities constructed after 1968 must meet the federal minimum standards for accessibility and usability. The Architectural and Transportation Barriers Compliance Board (A & TBCB) is the federal agency created to enforce the standards. Section 504 of the Rehabilitation Act of 1973 (effective date: June 3, 1977) provides that "no otherwise qualified handicapped individual shall, solely by reason of his handicap, be excluded from the participation in, be denied the benefits of, or be subjected to discrimination under any program or activity receiving federal financial assistance" (Non-discrimination on Basis of Handicap, 1977).

The implementation of these regulations requires change of attitude, financial support, and knowledge about the devices and standards available for establishing an accessible environment for people who have disabilities. There are various devices available that make an environment compatible with the capabilities of people with functional limitations.

Usry, Inc., recommends the following standard features for designing the home environment ("The Freedom Home"):

Standard Features

Minimum 4'0" width of hallway
No sills on exterior doors
All interior and exterior doors 36" wide with protector panels at bottom
Exterior doors with lever-operated door handles and two staggered door
    lights for outside viewing
Interior doors with lever operated handles
Window sills 2'4" off floor
Thermostats and electrical panel 48" from floor
Wall receptacles located 18" above floor
All switches touch control; located 48" above floor
Bi-fold door on bath for easy access
Special 5' × 6' shower
Single control handle on a safety water mixing valve for shower
Hand-held shower attachment
Grab bars in shower and at commode
Lavatory 31" high with long-reach mixer faucet, hand-held spray attach-
    ment, and large mirror above vanity
Open area under lavatory with insulated hot water lines
Master bedroom with easy access wardrobes and reachable clothes racks
Accessible kitchen with open area under sink and insulated hot water
    lines
Open area under counter-top range
Range hood with light
Built-in shelves on pantry door
Counter top 31" from floor
Overhead cabinets 12" above counters
Built-in electric oven with door that opens to counter height
Pull-down dinette light for easy bulb replacement

Barrier-free office buildings should be designed to include standards applicable to all disabilities. For blind persons, sound-reflecting walls are preferred. Other considerations for blind persons include steps and stairs without protruding nosings. This is also helpful for other ambulatory disabled and even nondisabled persons. Doors leading to dangerous areas, such as loading platforms, should be identified either with raised letters, with brailled lettering, or by use of textured flooring. Signals and signs should be communicated both audibly and visibly.

Standards for parking, curb cuts, ramps, door mechanisms, drinking fountains, floor coverings, space for wheelchair maneuvering, placement of windows, shelf height, height of wall telephones, and elevators switches are all important to consider. Reports such as "Building without Barriers for the Disabled" (Harkness and Groom, 1976), "Accessibility Modifications" (Mace, 1976), "A Design Guide for Home Safety" (1972), "An Illustrated Handbook of the Handicapped Section of the North Carolina State Building Code" (Mace and Iaslett, 1976), "Making Buildings and Facilities Accessible to and Usable by the Physically Handicapped" (1976), "Barrier Free Meetings" (Redden, 1976), "Home in a Wheelchair" (Chasin and Saltman, 1977), "Wheelchair Bathrooms" (Schweikert, 1977), and The National Center for a Barrier Free Environment provide standards for a barrier-free environment.

Modification of existing buildings is a common concern for many organizations. Commercially, many devices and information are available, a few of which are provided in the references (Handi-Ramp, Inc., Horton Automatics (Automatic Door); Power Access Corporation, "Automatic Door Opener, Model 4200"; Prentke Romich Company, "Remote Control Interior Door Operator for the Severely Handicapped"; Smith and Stevenson, Inc., "A Shower Stall for All People"; R-Anell Homes; Tubular Specialties Manufacturing, Inc., Catalog 785; Zuck and Eaton, Inc. (Patient Care Devices)). However, before installing devices or making major modifications, a qualified architect should be consulted regarding the most efficient and economical solution to a problem.

CONCLUSION

Information concerning many of the aids and devices mentioned in this chapter is available from the addresses listed in the reference lists. This chapter is not intended to provide evaluation of available items. However, any mentioned here is worthy of further investigation. Items produced by the Job Development Laboratory are mentioned for reference only. These are not commercially available, but if further information is desired concerning specific Job Development Laboratory items, please contact:

   The Job Development Laboratory
   Rehabilitation Research & Training Center
   The George Washington University
   2300 Eye St., N.W. Ross Hall 420
   Washington, D.C. 20037
   (202)676-3847

MANUFACTURERS/DISTRIBUTORS/ASSOCIATIONS

Accurate Medical Service
8004 Westchester Pike
Upper Darby, Pennsylvania 19082
(215) 259-3222

Accurate Medical Service
6630 U.S. Highway 130
Pennsauken, New Jersey 08109
(609) 665-3026

Alimed
138 Prince Street
Boston, Massachusetts 03113
(617) 227-0899

American Foundation for the Blind
15 West 16th Street
New York, New York 10011
(212) 924-0420

American Manufacturing Company,
   Inc.
2119 Pacific Avenue
Post Office Box 1237
Tacoma, Washington 98401

American Stair-Glide Corporation
4001 East 138 Street
Grandview, Missouri 64030

BARD/CARBA Division
731 Central Avenue
Murray Hill, New Jersey 07974

Bio Clinic Company
10507 Burbank Boulevard
North Hollywood, California 91601
(213) 985-4200

The Cheney Company
3015 South 163 Street
New Berlin, Wisconsin 53151
(404) 782-1100

Double Industries, Inc.
341 North Drive
St. Charles, Missouri 63301
(314) 946-3020

Down East Electronics Manufacturing
   Company
44 Bucknam Road
Falmouth, Maine 04105
(207) 774-9151

The Ealing Corporation
22 Pleasant Street
South Natick, Massachusetts 01760
(617) 655-7000

Earl's Stairway Lift Corporation
2513 Center Street
Cedar Falls, Iowa 50613
(319) 266-8878

Everest and Jennings, Inc.
1803 Pontius Avenue
Los Angeles, California 90025

EZMT Valve Company
Post Office Box 125
Mokena, Illinois 60448

Fidelity Electronics, Ltd.
5245 Diversey Avenue
Chicago, Illinois 60639
(312) 237-8090

G. E. Miller, Inc.
484 South Broadway
Yonkers, New York 10705

General Teleoperators, Inc.
Post Office Box 3584
Los Amigos Station
Downey, California 90242
(213) 923-4296

Gresham Driving Aids, Inc.
Post Office Box 405
30800 Wixom Road
Eixom, Michigan 48096
(313) 624-1533

Handi-Ramp, Inc.
1414 Armour Boulevard
Post Office Box 745
Mundelein, Illinois 60060
(312) 566-5861

Hausman Industries, Inc.
130 Union Street
Northvale, New Jersey 07647

HB & D Products
Post Office Box 743
South Laguna, California 92671
(714) 497-3139

Horton Automatics
6250 LB5 Freeway
Dallas, Texas 75204
(214) 233-6611

Innovations, Inc.
Post Office Box 1418-A
Pittsburg, Kansas 66762
(316) 231-1122

Institutional Industries
American Wheelchair Division
5500 Muddy Creek Road
Cincinnati, Ohio 45238

Intermed Associates, Inc.
39–41 Oak Ridge Road
New Foundland, New Jersey 07465
(201) 697-3373

Invacare Corporation
1200 Taylor Street
Elyria, Ohio 44035

J. A. Preston Corporation
71 Fifth Avenue
New York, New York 10023
(212) 255-8484

Lakeside Manufacturing, Inc.
1983 South Allis Street
Milwaukee, Wisonsin 53207
(414) 481-3900

Lumex, Inc.
100 Spence Street
Bayshore, New York 11706

Micon Industries
252 Oak Street
Oakland, California 94607
(415) 763-6033

National Center for Barrier Free
  Environment
8401 Connecticut Avenue, N.W.
Washington, D.C. 20015
(202) 656-9496

National Institute for Rehabilitation
  Engineering
59 Hamburg Turnpike
Pompton Lakes, New Jersey 07442

National Railroad Passenger Access
  AMTRAK
955 L'Enfant Plaza, S. W.
Washington, D.C. 20024

Para Industries, Ltd.
6-4826 11th Street, N.E.
Calgary, Alberta T2E2W7, Canada
(403) 276-3133

Pew Memorial Trust Fund
Services for the Blind
919 Walnut Street
Philadelphia, Pennsylvania 19107

PMV System AA-MED, Inc.
1215 S. Harlem Ave.
Forest Park, Illinois 60130
(312) 626-1500

Power Access Corporation
96 Birch Avenue
Little Silver, New Jersey 07739

Prentke Romich Company
R.D. 2, Post Office Box 191
Shreve, Ohio 44676
(216) 567-2906

R-Anell Homes
Route 2, Post Office Box 71
Maxton, North Carolina 28364
(919) 844-5055

Romich, Beery and Bayer, Inc.
R.D. 2, Post Office Box 191
Shreve, Ohio 44676
(216) 567-2906

Scope Electronics, Inc.
1860 Michael Faraday Drive
Reston, Virginia 22090
(703) 471-5600

Smith and Stevenson, Inc.
Post Office Box 15008
Charlotte, North Carolina 28210
(704) 525-3388

Stanley Door Operating Equipment
  Division
Farmington, Connecticut 06032
(203) 677-2861

Talley Surgical Instruments, Ltd.
47 Theobald Street
Borehamwood Herts, England
Distributed by: HAAG Brothers, Inc.
2920 North Arlington Heights Road
Arlington Heights, Illinois 60004
(312) 394-2700

Ted Hoyer & Company, Inc.
2222 Minnesota Street
Oshkosh, Wisconsin 54901
Distributed by: Everest and Jennings
1803 Pontius Avenue
Los Angeles, California 90025

Telesensory Systems, Inc.
1889 Page Mill Road
Palo Alto, California 94304

Thomas Built Buses, Inc.
1408 Courtesy Road
Highpoint, North Carolina 27261

Toce Brothers Manufacturing, Ltd.
Post Office Box 489
Broussard, Louisiana 70518
(318) 856-5941

Touch Turner Company
1808 Tenth Avenue
East Seattle, Washington 98102
(206) 323-7534

Triaxon, Inc.
Post Office Box 415
Glenview, Illinois 60025
(312) 724-0038

Tubular Specialties Manufacturing,
   Inc.
8119 South Beach Street
Post Office Box 71527
Florence Branch
Los Angeles, California 90001
(213) 583-4931

Usry, Inc.
Post Office Box 27463
1415 Chamberlane Avenue
Richmond, Virginia 23261
(804) 321-4500

Viking
Post Office Box 318
Middlebury, Indiana 45640
(219) 825-8401

Visualtek
1610 26th Street
Santa Monica, California 90404
(213) 829-3453

The Wheelchair Carrier Corporation
5829 North Seventh Street
Post Office Box 9328
Phoenix, Arizona 85268
(602) 265-5666

Zuck and Eaton, Inc.
Medical Equipment and Supplies
1696 Northrock Drive
Rockford, Illinois 61103
(815) 877-1411

REFERENCES

Annand, D. R. 1971. The wheelchair traveler. D. R. Annand, Milford, N.H.
Architectural and Transportation Barriers Compliance Board. 1977. Access America: The architectural barriers act and you. Washington, D.C.
Brown, E. B. 1975. Independent mobility and the disabled. In K. Mallik, S. Yuspeh, and J. Mueller (eds.), Comprehensive Vocational Rehabilitation for Severely Disabled Persons. Job Development Laboratory, Washington, D.C.
Chasin, J., and Saltman, J. 1977. Home in a wheelchair. Paralyzed Veterans of America, Inc., Washington, D.C.
A design guide for home safety. 1972. U.S. Department of Housing and Urban Development, Washington, D.C.

The handicapped majority and aids for the handicapped. 1974. Industrial Design 21(4):22–45.

Harkness, S. P., and Groom, J. N. 1976. Building without barriers for the disabled. Watson-Guptill Publications, New York.

Howard, G. 1975. Helping the handicapped: A guide to aids. Telephone Pioneers of America, New York.

Jamero, P. 1976. Eliminate mobility barriers, employ rehabilitants. Division of Vocational Rehabilitation, Olympia, Wash.

Kafafian, H. 1970. Study of Man-Machine Communication Systems for the Handicapped. Vol. I and II. Cybernetics Research Institute, Washington, D.C.

Kafafian, H. 1973. Study of Man-Machine Communication Systems for the Handicapped. Vol. III. Cybernetics Research Institute, Washington, D.C.

Kliment, S. A. 1975. Into the mainstream—A syllabus for a barrier free environment. The American Institute of Architects, Washington, D.C.

Leslie, J., Shute, C. T., Norris, R. H., and Moss, J. L. 1976. Development of comprehensive competitive employment services for the physically handicapped—Phase II Report. Wichita State University, College of Engineering, Wichita.

Lowman, E., and Klinger, J. L. 1969. Aids to independent living: Self help for the handicapped. McGraw-Hill Book Company, New York.

Low vision service. 1974. The New York Association for the Blind, New York.

Mace, R. I. 1976. Accessibility modifications. Barrier Free Environments, Inc., Raleigh, N.C.

Mace, R. I., and Iaslett, B. 1976. An illustrated handbook of the handicapped section of the North Carolina state building code. Governor's Committee on Architectural Barriers and Department of Insurance, N.C.

Macey, P. G. 1974. Mobilizing multiply handicapped children: A manual for the design and construction of modified wheelchairs. University of Kansas, Lawrence.

Making buildings and facilities accessible to and usable by the physically handicapped. 1976. Syracuse University School of Architecture Research Office, Syracuse, N.Y.

Mallik, K. 1975. Vocational direction through information handling technology. Comprehensive Vocational Rehabilitation for Severely Disabled Persons. The Job Development Laboratory, Washington, D.C.

Mallik, K., and Mueller, J. 1975. Vocational aids and enchanced productivity of the severely disabled. Proceedings of Systems and Devices for the Disabled 2:203–207.

Mallik, K., and Mueller, J. 1977. A practical design approach to rehabilitation products. Proceedings of Systems and Devices for the Disabled 4:A36–A39.

Mallik, K., and Sablowsky, R. Models for placement—Job laboratory approach. J. Rehab. 42(6):14–21.

Mallik, K., and Shworles, T. 1971. A simple adaptation on modern vocational tools bring new work opportunities for the homebound. Rehab. Gazette 14:46–50.

Mallik, K., Shaver, E., High, E., and Mueller, J. 1977. Communications for the developmentally disabled: A resource guide for parents and professionals. The Job Development Laboratory, Washington, D.C.

Mallik, K., and Yuspeh, S. 1975. Bio-engineering services to the developmentally disabled adolescent. The Job Development Laboratory, Washington, D.C.

McCluer, S., Conry, J. E., Gephardt, S. L., Rice, W., and Wike, R. 1974. Assistive devices and equipment for rehabilitation. Arkansas Rehabilitation Research and Training Center, Hot Spring.

Melichar, O. 1975. Information system on adaptive, assistive and recreational equipment, ISAARE, Vol. I–VI. United Cerebral Palsy Association, Portland, Or.

Nickerson, R. S., and Stevens, K. N. Using computers to help deaf children to speak. Science, Technology and the Handicapped Report #76R11. American Association for the Advancement of Science, Washington, D.C.

Non-discrimination on basis of handicap. 1977. Federal Register.

Optical Aids Service—Survey. 1957. Industrial Home for the Blind, Brooklyn.

Product/Service Buyer's Guide for the Rehabilitation Industries. 1976. Green Pages, Winter Park, Fla.

Redden, M. 1976. Barrier free meetings: A guide for professional associations. American Association for the Advancement of Science, Washington, D.C.

Robinault, I. P. 1973. Functional aids for the multiply handicapped. Harper & Row Publishers, New York.

Shweikert, H. A. Jr. 1977. Wheelchair bathrooms. Paralyzed Veterans of America, Inc., Washington, D.C.

Shworles, T., and Mallik, K. 1971a. New productive capability and earnings of physically disabled homebound persons. J. Micrograph. 4(4):223–231.

Shworles, T., and Mallik, K. 1971b. Technological change and new vocational opportunities for homebound severely disabled persons. Int. Assoc. Rehab. Facil. 201–213.

Sullivan, R. A., Frieden, F. H., and Corder, J. 1968. Telephone services for the handicapped. Rehab. Monogr. XXXVII. Institute of Rehabilitation Medicine, New York, University Medical Center, New York.

TSI's computer now reads. 1977. TSI Newsletter #15. Talley Surgical Instruments, Borehamwood Herts, England.

United Cerebral Palsy Association. 1975. Information Systems on Adaptive Assistive Recreational Equipment 1–6.

Vanderheiden, G. C., and Grilley, K. 1975. Non-vocal communication techniques and aids for the severely physically handicapped. University Park Press, Baltimore.

Chapter 9

What Happens After Placement? Career Enhancement Services in Vocational Rehabilitation

Dennis J. Dunn

Editor's note: The emphasis on placement has become so paramount within rehabilitation that long-range career development has often been neglected. This chapter is one of the few sources that explores the post-placement or career enhancement phase of career development within the rehabilitation process. To date, little conceptual work has been done and few practical approaches are available to guide planning for career enhancement after placement occurs.

Preparing for a job, securing one, and then pursuing a career are three distinct processes requiring different knowledge and skills. In order to offer career development opportunities to clients, rehabilitation services must attend to each of these areas and specific planning and services must be implemented for each.

This chapter provides a way to start developing a conceptual approach to client-oriented, career enhancement rehabilitation services. Practical approaches are offered for use within the context of rehabilitation service delivery. Many of these approaches require counseling expertise, which suggests that persons involved in placement and career follow-up should be capable of counseling; this issue cannot be ignored when educating rehabilitation professionals.

This chapter is only a beginning. More emphasis must be given to this area in rehabilitation research and practice. In particular, employer-oriented, as well as client-oriented, career enhancement must be explained.

A major problem in the delivery of post-placement services is the lack of understanding about what is to be included in them. The conceptual framework determining the provision of vocational rehabilitation services preceding placement is reasonably well defined, as are the services typically necessary to achieve this goal. This is not true in the case of post-placement services. The conceptual framework has not been well defined, nor have typical services been identified.

The purpose to this chapter is to develop a conceptual framework for post-placement services. This is based to a great extent on information available on the career development of persons without disabilities. A second purpose is to identify problem areas that are likely to be encountered by persons with disabilities and to suggest intervention strategies and techniques designed to deal with these problems.

AN OVERVIEW OF POST-PLACEMENT SERVICES

Much time and effort have been devoted to defining such terms as *placement services*, *placement process*, and *post-placement services* and to determining who does what to whom. In this chapter, placement is defined as an *event* that occurs when an individual has accepted a job offer that will yield appropriate career development opportunities (Vandergoot, Jacobsen, and Worrall, 1978). This view is in contrast to the traditional view, which implies that placement is an event marking the *end point* of the rehabilitation process. This definition recognizes placement as the *beginning point* of a nontraditional vocational rehabilitation process. Ultimately, this process should ensure the attainment of available career development opportunities for the worker.

"Career development is a process which people use, over the extent of their lives, to receive the financial and nonmonetary reward from society which they desire" (Vandergoot, Jacobsen, and Worrall, 1978, p. 15). More specifically, *career development* refers to "the lifelong process of developing work, values, crystallizing a vocational identity, learning about opportunities, and trying out plans in part time, recreational, and full time work situations" (Tolbert, 1974, p. 25). Career development is often viewed strictly in occupational terms; that is, as a sequence of occupations, jobs, and positions that have a common theme and a steady upward progression in responsibility, earnings, status, and personal satisfaction. Many careers follow this kind of growth pattern (Crites, 1969; Slocum, 1966). Others do not. For some people, career development is a process of personal growth and development in relation to a stable occupation or employment situation (Levinson et al., 1978). These individuals show growth and maturation of work values and vocational identities which enable them to fully appreciate working, even in occupations that others might view as undesirable or uninteresting. The common thread in career development, whether it is achieved by occupational advancement, by personal growth, or by some combination of the two, is that it is an active process—one that involves coping, adapting, planning, and taking risks (Kroll et al., 1970). As conceived in the first chapter, career development consists of three phases: 1) productivity enrichment, 2) productivity realization, and 3) career enhancement.

Nested within the phase of career enhancement is *work establishment*, the process by which an individual achieves "attachment to an occupation in an organization, stability of employment and minimum protection against risk, and earnings sufficient to enable the worker to support himself and his dependents according to accepted standards of health and decency" (Freedman, 1969, p. 5). Work establishment refers to the process of "settling in" to the labor force (Ornstein, 1976). Attachments are formed within the labor force, identity as a worker is established and shaped, and errors in the selection of the initial job are corrected. The process may involve changing jobs more than once (with each change requiring a new "work adjustment") and typically requires about 3 to 5 years to achieve. Work establishment basically means making a transition into work and the labor force and developing commitments.

Work adjustment is a process that recurs throughout the entire career cycle. Lofquist and Dawis (1969) define work adjustment as "the continuous and dynamic process by which the individual seeks to achieve and maintain correspondence with his work environment" (p. 46). The basic mechanisms by which work adjustment is achieved are described in the Minnesota Theory of Work Adjustment. This theory deals with the problems involved in coping with and adapting to the specific work environments surrounding particular jobs and positions. Each time an individual changes position a new adjustment is called for. Ordinarily, within vocational rehabilitation, work adjustment is a type of service program offered by rehabilitation facilities to clients with basic limitations in employability such as problems in attendance, punctuality, co-worker and supervisory relationships, and so on. The Minnesota Theory does not view work adjustment as a service program, however, but a process that can continue throughout the working life of the individual.

Career enhancement may best be viewed as the broad process that subsumes the two others. Work establishment is the initial part of the career enhancement process. Unless the worker successfully enters the labor force, establishing an identity as a worker and verifying the choices related to career theme and occupation, career development cannot continue. Similarly, work adjustment occurs throughout a worker's entire career. Work adjustment failures that take place early in the work

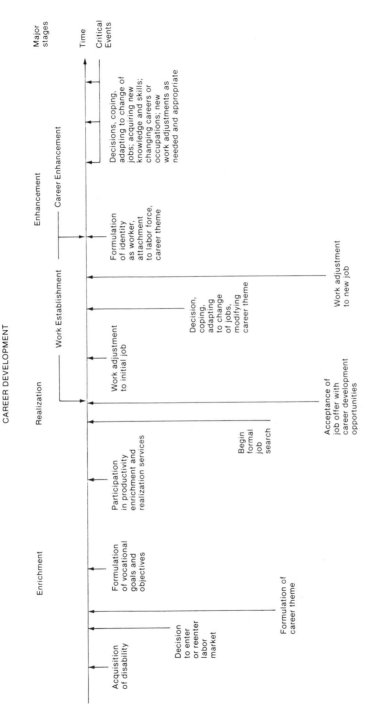

Figure 1. Major stages and critical events in the career development process of persons with disabilities.

establishment stage would adversely affect the work establishment process. This in turn would affect the entire career process, making early adjustments critical to successful work establishment.

The overall relationships between the career development phases, as they occur within a rehabilitation process, and critical events that occur along a hypothetical timeline are shown in Figure 1. This is, of course, an oversimplification of a complex set of events but it does provide a picture of what occurs over time, beginning with the onset of disability. Moreover, examining critical events makes it clear that the early part of the rehabilitation process, particularly handling issues related to coping and adapting to disability, and vocational decision-making, have direct analogs later in career enhancement. In a practical sense, the rehabilitation process is a learning experience in which skills and behaviors necessary for later career enhancement are acquired and mastered.

The balance of this chapter provides a more detailed discussion of career enhancement and its basic processes. The conceptual and empirical material related to each process are presented first, followed by a discussion of intervention techniques that could be used to deal with problems.

WORK ADJUSTMENT

The central concept in the Minnesota Theory of Work Adjustment is that of correspondence. Correspondence involves satisfactoriness and satisfaction. Satisfactoriness, typically considered in vocational rehabilitation, refers to the congruence between the individual's abilities and the performance requirements of the position. If there is a critical minimum level of correspondence, the individual will be perceived as competent by the employer and will be retained on the job or promoted.

The satisfaction dimension has not been stressed to any great extent in vocational rehabilitation. It refers to the congruence between the individual's needs and the reinforcers available in the work environment that will satisfy these needs. If there is a critical minimum level of correspondence between needs and reinforcers, the individual will perceive the environment as satisfying and will remain on the job.

Tenure, or the length of stay on the job, is a function of *both* satisfactoriness and satisfaction. It reflects the fact that employers and employees both make demands of each other. Employers have performance demands and employees have reinforcer demands. Unless both sets of demands are met, the individual will be fired, transferred, or will quit.

The relationships between the various dimensions in the Minnesota Theory of Work Adjustment are shown in Figure 2. The dashed lines in

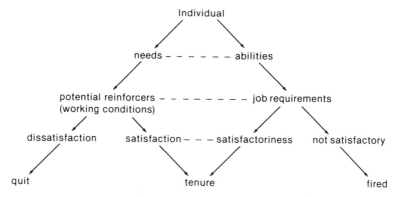

Figure 2. Schematic of the Minnesota Theory of Work Adjustment.

the figure represent moderator effects, in which satisfactoriness can affect satisfaction and vice versa. For example, assume an individual with a high need for money is working on a piecework job. If there is correspondence between the individual's abilities and the job requirements, the rates can be met or exceeded so that the need for money is met. The individual would be both satisfactory and satisfied, with the degree of satisfaction depending partially on the degree of satisfactoriness. Conversely, if the individual's abilities were not correspondent with the requirements set by piece rates, less money would be received, leading to a decrease in satisfaction. These moderator effects have not been sufficiently studied, but they may be extremely important in understanding the work adjustment process.

Within natural work environments, reinforcement is often contingent upon complex communication chains within small work groups (Staats and Staats, 1963), which is another potential moderator. The individual's responses serve as stimuli for responses made by other members of the group. Similarly, the authority of a supervisor is partly contingent upon the type of stimuli presented by the individual, which initiates an authority sequence (Staats and Staats, 1963).

It is beyond the scope of this chapter to analyze these communication chains in any detail. Additional material can be found in texts such as Staats and Staats (1963) or Karen (1974). The point to keep in mind is that an inability to engage in required social interactions with co-workers and supervisors can affect *both* satisfactoriness (since ability requirements are not met) and satisfaction (since reinforcers under the control of co-workers or supervisors are not delivered).

Two ideas were introduced in the preceding paragraphs that need some elaboration. The first is that abilities and ability requirements include things that are usually labeled "behaviors." The second is that reinforcement of behavior comes from co-workers as well as supervisors.

Abilities and Ability Requirements

The use of the term *ability* within the Minnesota Theory of Work Adjustment and the measurement of ability using the General Aptitude Test Battery in research on the theory is unfortunate. It brings to mind the psychometric concept of ability and notions of traits. Dawis (1976) has clarified the meaning of the term within the context of the theory. He notes that work is organized "into more or less standard sets of tasks (required behaviors) called jobs (or more precisely, positions)." People hired for a job are presumably capable of performing it; "in more technical terms, they have the behavior, or response, capabilities for the job." Furthermore, "response capabilities, when categorized into a smaller number of classes, are what might be called *abilities*. A person utilizes abilities to meet the behavior requirements . . . of a job" (Dawis, 1976, p. 231). Abilities, therefore, reflect a person's performance of job-relevant behaviors.

Within the Minnesota Theory of Work Adjustment, abilities and ability requirements are general categories of response capabilities and response requirements. From a theoretical point of view, a generalized concept of abilities and ability requirements is convenient when describing the behavior of a group of persons dealing with a job (or group of similar jobs in several establishments). Generalization may be an inconvenience or may even impede the application of the theory when an individual worker is adjusting to a specific position because it can obscure the details of correspondence between the individual's specific response capabilities and the behavioral requirements of the position.

Role of Co-workers

Work is seldom performed in isolation. More typically it is performed by small work groups in which workers perform unique sets of tasks on an object in linear fashion (as in an assembly line) or a similar set of tasks concurrently (as in a word processing center). This organization tends to promote interactions among members of the work group. The group itself can be a source of strength, encouragement, and reinforcement to the worker. Conversely, it can be the source of unhappiness or even a reason for a worker to leave an otherwise suitable job.

The Hawthorne studies were among the first to establish that work groups controlled the behavior of the individual members (Roethlisberger and Dickson, 1940). Roy's (1952) study of machine shop workers demonstrated how the production norms of a work group were at variance with those established by management. In a subsequent study, he described ritualistic joking and other interaction patterns among these workers (Roy, 1960).

Braude (1975) has described in some detail how membership in work groups is typically attained by successfully "passing" a series of initiation rites. Some of these can be humbling or even demeaning to the individual. Once passed, however, the new worker is advanced to "colleagueship" and is entitled to the protection of the group. Braude (1975) views the induction process as one that results in a sense of identity for the worker.

For the new worker, the existence of the work group with its particular set of behavioral requirements and demands poses a significant challenge. The worker must not only meet the demands established by management, but also those set up by the work group. To adjust, the worker must make a compromise by which the major demands of both groups are satisfactorily met. Dealing only with the needs of one group while ignoring those of the other can be disastrous for the individual. Even after membership in the work group has been attained, the worker must continually juggle actual behavior to meet the sometimes conflicting expectations of the work group and management. Although horseplay is frowned on by management, it may be required by the group, and although high productivity may be valued by management, it may be frowned on by the group.

Stress, Coping, and Adaptation

Although Lofquist and Dawis (1969) define work adjustment as a "continuous and dynamic process," the process has not been adequately described or researched. However, Dawis and Lofquist (1976) and Dawis (1976) have postulated a set of four personality style dimensions that may affect the work adjustment process. These are described in Table 1, along with hypothesized clinical indicators, which could be obtained from a review of historical data sources as well as observation of behavior.

The first dimension, flexibility, determines the zone of discorrespondence that can be tolerated before it becomes unmanageable and causes the individual to leave the environment. This can be subdivided into an "area of tolerable discorrespondence" and an "area of adjustment" (Dawis and Lofquist, 1976). When the individual's level of correspondence is within the area of adjustment, the person will change the work environment (active response) or the work personality (reactive response), which are the second and third dimensions. The fourth dimension, celerity, determines the rate at which these changes will take place.

Dawis (1976) suggests that similar dimensions may be used to describe the way in which the work environment accommodates an individual. In other words, organizations may vary in the degree to which

Table 1. Personality styles and their clinical indicators

Personality dimension	Definition	Clinical indicators	
		High level	Low level
Flexibility	The degree to which an individual can tolerate discorrespondence with the work environment	Participation in a wide range of situations Experience in a wide range of situations Successful work history in a wide range of jobs Heterogeneous group of friends	Participation in a narrow range of activities Exposure to a narrow range of situations Narrow range of successful jobs Limited or homogeneous group of friends
Activeness	The degree to which the individual acts on the work environment to increase correspondence with the work personality	Has held positions of leadership Organized groups and activities Developed new ways of doing things Has taken initiative in school, work, or community activities	Lack of initiative Lack of innovativeness

Reactiveness	The degree to which the individual changes the work personality to increase correspondence with the work environment	History of abiding by the rules Carries out assignments according to prescribed procedures Comfort/satisfaction in structured groups/situations Participation as member, not leader, of group	Inability to participate in group situations Difficulty in following rules and prescribed procedures Social isolation
Rate of adjustment (Celerity)	The rate of movement toward increased correspondence	Prompt/early completion of assignments Almost impulsive behavior Emphasizing speed of response over accuracy.	Deliberateness of response Apparent procrastination Long response latencies

Adapted from Lofquist and Dawis (1976).

they can tolerate discorrespondent individuals (flexibility), their response style (active or reactive), and their rate of response (celerity). One could hypothesize that a set of "clinical indicators" similar to Table 1 could be developed for specific jobs within a given organization. For example, flexibility might be indicated by differences in duties and tasks assigned to positions within a job classification; activeness by the degree to which training and other experiences are provided to increase the correspondence of individuals with the work environment; reactivity by the degree to which the organization makes changes in assigned duties and tasks to accommodate the response capabilities of individual employees; and celerity by the rate at which training or position modification responses are made. This formulation suggests that there would be a reciprocal relationship between personal and organizational response styles, with individuals having an active personal response style doing best in reactive organizations and vice versa.

French, Rodgers, and Cobb (1974), in their analysis of person-environment fit, point out the differences between objectively measured and subjectively perceived reports of individual abilities and needs as well as environmental demands and reinforcers. The fit between a person and the environment can be described objectively and subjectively. *Reality contact* can be described as the congruence between objective and subjective reports of environmental characteristics, while *accuracy of person assessment* can be described as the congruence between objective and subjective personal characteristics. In situations where there is discorrespondence, or lack of objective fit, the individual can *cope* by making objective changes or can *defend* by making subjective changes without corresponding objective changes.

The importance of the French et al. (1974) model lies in its inclusion of subjective perceptions in the definition of person-environment fit. The Minnesota Theory of Work Adjustment deals exclusively with the objective correspondence between individuals and their work environments. Subjective correspondence is equally as important to consider, particularly in the case of persons with disabilities as they enter or reenter the labor force. The way they perceive environmental demands, especially when these include the initiation rites imposed upon all new workers in the setting, may decrease reality contact with the environment. Similarly, Korman's (1970, 1971) research into the relationship among expectations of others, task performance, and self-assessment suggests that the accuracy of self-assessment may decline if significant others within the work environment have stereotyped negative expectations about the person because of a disability.

When entering a new job, the individual confronts a set of major adaptive tasks that must be performed.[1] Some of these are related directly to the job itself and are: 1) dealing with the performance demands of the job, 2) dealing with the work and organizational environment, 3) developing adequate relationships with co-workers and supervisors, and 4) dealing with increased responsiblities and demands within the community. Others are general in nature and involve maintenance of existing functions. These include: 1) maintaining emotional stability, 2) maintaining accurate self-perception, and 3) maintaining relationships with family and friends. Acquiring a job upsets the individual's equilibrium; it creates a stressful situation, increasing tension and anxiety. The extent to which the individual experiences stress and eventually crisis depends on the demands of the environment and the individual's capacity to deal with them. If the worker possesses adequate coping skills to resolve a particular problem situation, the stressful experience is resolved successfully. If, however, existing coping skills are not adequate, the situation becomes a crisis. Crises involve long-term stress and must be resolved by some type of permanent change in the individual's personality organization or response repertoire. The acquisition of new coping skills enables the individual to successfully resolve the problems. It is possible for no learning or for inappropriate learning to occur. In both of these situations, since the problem is not successfully dealt with, the individual would continue to experience disorganization and crisis.

Figure 3 summarizes this discussion and shows how stress, crisis, and adaptation are interrelated. Underlying this model is the idea that basic learning principles apply to stress and its resolution. In other words, stress can be resolved by applying existing knowledge and skills to the problem. If established knowledge and skills do not help, acquiring necessary ways of coping must occur before the crisis ends.

Intervention in Work Adjustment

During the past decade a number of intervention techniques appropriate to dealing with problems in work adjustment have been developed. Some derive from the extensive amount of work done by the Department of Labor in placement of disadvantaged and minority group members. Other techniques have been developed within the field of behavior modification, particularly by researchers closely associated with social learning approaches.

Intervention can be viewed as having two dimensions: prevention and treatment. Prevention involves things like developing requisite

---

[1] This discussion is adapted from Moos and Tsu (1977).

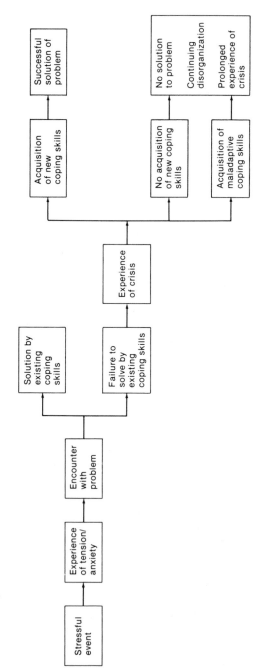

Figure 3.   Stress and its resolution. (Adapted from Kroll et al., 1970, p. 187.)

knowledge, skills, and other behavior before placement and structuring and arranging the immediate environment to preclude or minimize the development of adjustment problems once the person is working.

Prevention   A fundamental prevention strategy is to make use of models. Bandura (1969, 1971, 1977) has drawn attention to the central role of models in the acquisition of new social behavior. The observation of an appropriately functioning model within the work environment indicates to the new worker both the expected behaviors within the setting and the consequences of their reinforcement. As Bandura (1977) points out: "The capacity to learn by observation enables people to acquire large, integrated patterns of behavior without having to form them by tedious trial and error." Modeling can be facilitated by the use of a buddy system. Hershenson (1974) describes this as assigning the new employee to an experienced co-worker with a similar disability. The buddy aids in the adjustment to work by serving as a model and providing direct assistance. It may not always be possible to find another worker with a disability to function as a buddy, but it usually is possible to find a member of the work group who would be willing to serve this role of helping the new worker "learn the ropes." In fact, within many informal work groups, one member already has this helping role. It may be necessary to teach individuals how to deal comfortably with a person who has a disability. Once done, however, there can be benefits in work adjustment beyond those described earlier. If the new employee is perceived as the buddy, or more correctly the protégé, of an established member of the work group, it may be easier for the worker to become a group member. Braude (1975) has indicated that group membership is a crucial step in the long-term work adjustment of the individual.

Burke, Weir, and Duncan (1976) have investigated helping and supportive relationships between workers in an organization. They found that a considerable amount of helping took place, mostly in relationship to problems about work procedures, policies, assignments, and working relationships. The helping interaction was most commonly initiated by the person in need of help and usually resulted in the problem either being resolved or else being clarified with movement made toward attaining a solution. They concluded that assistance provided by group members was an important means of solving work-related problems encountered by workers.

Job coaches are the center of another preventive strategy. The coach is an agency employee responsible for assisting the client "in such things as learning how to get to work, learning to be prompt and reliable, learning how to do the job tasks, and learning how to budget . . . wages" (Hershenson, 1974, p. 494). The coach can serve a valuable function during the initial adjustment period by identifying and solving problems before they become crises for the individual, the employer, or the work group.

A third and underused preventive strategy is the creation of both professional and self-help groups to assist persons with disabilities in making a satisfactory work adjustment. Azrin and his associates have shown the effectiveness of professionally run groups in assisting individuals to find jobs (Azrin, Flores, and Kaplan, 1975), while Stuart (1977) has reviewed the effectiveness of self-help groups in assisting individuals to successfully deal with a variety of behavior problems.

Although some VR agencies and rehabilitation facility programs have made use of follow-up group counseling (Hershenson, 1974), detailed behavioral analyses similar to those underlying Azrin's Job Finding Club program model have not been conducted to date. Although the leading cause of work adjustment failure is believed to be interpersonal problems, there are no empirical data to support this belief, nor is there a detailed analysis available about interpersonal problems that could form the foundation of a Job Keeping Club program model for professional or self-help groups.

Treatment   Treatment approaches exist for many of the specific problems individuals encounter during work adjustment. Assuming that behavior in interpersonal situations is a fundamental problem, consideration could be given to behavior rehearsal (Goldfried and Davison, 1976), an approach shown to be effective in training individuals to assume a new behavioral role, such as that of a worker. To be effective, however, behavior rehearsal requires that the counselor have detailed knowledge of the specific role expectations held by others within the client's work environment. This type of environmental analysis is typically neglected. It is similar to the job analysis that is done to establish job duties, tasks, and performance requirements, and it may be more important to the ultimate success of the individual than a job analysis. Behavior rehearsal is commonly done in a one-to-one helping situation. Rose (1977) points out, however, that there is no reason why it cannot be done in a group, and provides specific illustrations of behavior rehearsal in group settings.

The model for work adjustment presented earlier in this section suggests that problems in the areas of stress management, anxiety control, and problem solving may be more central in work adjustment failure than the current literature suggests. Deficiencies in the area of problem solving can be dealt with by assisting the individual to acquire essential problem-solving skills (Goldfried and Davison, 1976). Similarly, Meichenbaum's (1977) stress innoculation training approach can be used to assist individuals in acquiring effective means of coping with stressful situations. This approach combines systematic desensitization, modeling, and self-instructional training. Anxiety is perhaps the most common human problem and, as Bernstein (1976) has pointed out, may not be a unitary construct, but rather a label that encompasses a variety of responses. Anxiety is one of the most extensively studied problems and numerous approaches to its management have been developed. These include relaxation training, systematic desensitization, and the cognitive relabeling and restructuring approaches (Goldfried and Davison, 1976). All these methods can be used in both group and individual settings (Rose, 1977).

The successful adjustment of an individual to a work setting may involve treating the existing work group as well as the person. Placing an individual with a disability into a work group can create anxiety or disrupt patterns of interpersonal interaction. It was noted earlier in this section that the work setting is dynamic and change in one part of the system can affect other parts, perhaps in unknown ways. The targets for post-employment services during the work adjustment phase may be members of the work group, a supervisor, or a manager. Alteration of their behavior *toward* the individual with a disability can have a reciprocal effect on the behavior shown by that individual in the work setting. Burke et al. (1976), in their study of informal helping relationships, found that the helping activities that occurred tended to be problem- and action-centered, rather than person-centered and concerned with the feelings and emotions of others. An implication of this is that co-workers and supervisors may need assistance and training in the use of listening, empathy, and support as helping behaviors.

In summary, the technology exists to permit successful intervention into those problems that can reasonably be expected to occur during periods of work adjustment. The harsh conclusion to be drawn from that fact is that failure is not so much the fault of clients or of nasty, insensitive people within work environments as it is of the failure of rehabilitation workers to identify potential and actual problems and to use the existing technology to resolve them. Intervention will not be successful in every case: the complexities of human behavior work against that. However intervention in the form of both prevention and treatment can be used more than it is currently to deal with work adjustment problems. The state of the art does not even permit a descriptive listing of the significant problems encountered by persons with disabilities once they start their jobs. This, in itself, is indicative of the lack of attention to work adjustment concerns.

WORK ESTABLISHMENT

Work establishment has been defined as a settling-in process in which a worker acquires an attachment to an organization or occupation, achieves stable and protected employment, improves earnings, and corrects errors in initial job selection (Freedman, 1969; Ornstein, 1976). The process of work establishment covers a 3- to 5-year period during which the worker makes a transition into work. Oddly enough, even though the adequacy of this transition can have a tremendous impact upon subsequent career behavior, and most theories of career development recognize such things as transition and trial (Super, 1957), there have been very few studies of the work establishment process. Those that have been done have focused upon the entry and work establishment behavior of males and females as a general group (Freedman, 1969; Ornstein, 1976; Parnes et al., 1976; Kohen et al., 1977). The work establishment behavior of persons with disabilities has not been specifically studied.

The most striking finding of the work establishment research is the extent and degree to which job-changing occurs. Ornstein (1976) found that "6 out of 10 white respondents and 4 out of 10 black respondents change(d) jobs" in the first 2 years after entering the labor force. Job-changing after entry commonly involves major shifts in both occupation and industry. Freedman (1969) found that more than three-quarters of all changes involved an occupational change, while 87% involved a change in industry. Kohen et al. (1977) had similar findings; about two-thirds of their sample had changed major occupational groups during the first 6 years after entry. The proportions of individuals changing occupations varied considerably according to the occupational group of the first job. For example, 77% of those white males who entered the labor force in the professional and technical occupational group stayed in it, compared with only 11% of those who entered in the non-farm laboring occupational group. White male laborers were most likely to have shown upward occupational mobility into the operative (36%) and craft (25%) occupational groups.

Kohen et al. (1977) attempted to explain the likelihood of advancement using a prediction model based upon factors such as formal education, vocational training, veteran status, occupational information, and so on. Although significant regression coefficients were obtained for most of these variables, the overall regression model could only account for approximately one-third of the variance observed. This finding led Kohen et al. (1977) to suggest that "there is a large component of randomness in the occupational mobility of new labor market participants" (p. 124). They do point out, however, that even though there is

> a significant degree of random 'milling around' among occupations, industries, and employers . . . it should be recognized that some of the milling around that typifies the establishment of career thresholds is, nonetheless, functional in terms of providing labor market information upon which later mobility may be more 'rationally' based (Kohen et al., 1977, p. 95).

Kohen et al. (1977) also examined all of the job separations that occurred to the men in the sample within a single year. Most of the separations were voluntary, made up of individuals who either found another job before quitting the current one (25.2%) or who did not (28.2%). Of those who quit without a prearranged job, the leading causes of leaving were dislike of hours or conditions (54.7%), closely followed by personal or family reasons (23.2%).

The job separation data give some indication of the adverse impact of health and disability on labor force participation. Kohen et al. (1977) included separation for health and disability reasons in their "low volition" category; i.e., "those separations involving little or no volition on the part of the worker." Low volition separations accounted for 40.9% of all separations. Table 2 shows the subsequent labor force participation rates of these individuals. Among males 19 to 29 years old, 34% of the individuals separated for health or disability reasons withdrew from the labor force altogether. Disability occurring within the establishment period appears to have a major negative impact upon the worker's subsequent labor force participation.

Occupational mobility, whether measured by status or wages, tends to depend upon the educational level of the individual and the occupational level of the job at entry. These factors and others are statistically related to occupational mobility, but not to the extent to which they could be used to reliably estimate mobility in individual cases. Examining the mobility of new workers, Freedman (1969) found that *within* given firms, worker characteristics were generally poor predictors of mobility. Organizational variables are better predictors of mobility. The technical level and diversity of the tasks necessary for continued maintenance of the firm were a fundamental factor. Mobility is maximized in those firms that have a diverse internal labor market with complex occupational ladders. These provide constantly increasing technical skill levels that

Table 2.   Subsequent labor force participation for low volition job separation

| | | | Labor force participation | | | |
| | Total | | Remained | | Left | |
Reason for separation	N	%	N	%	N	%
Layoff, plant closed, end of temporary job (laid off and recalled)	520 (72)	80	520 (72)	100 (100)	0 (0)	0 (0)
Discharged	43	7	42	93	3	7
Health or disability	47	7	31	66	16	34
Closed own business	42	6	38	90	4	10

Adapted from Kohen et al. (1977), Table 5.9.

employees can attain. A second major organizational factor had to do with promotional style. Mobility is maximized in those firms that have objective promotional systems based on testing, and in those firms that have formal, job-related, company-sponsored training programs. The third major factor involved the presence of "purely organizational upgrading." This factor essentially reflects the degree to which the firm can retitle or reclassify existing jobs to produce higher status and pay for workers within them.

Freedman's (1969) study indicated that "establishment takes place through filling an organizational position" (p.112). This is somewhat different than the usual concept of establishment, which tends to be occupationally based on and formulated from the idea of worker characteristics being the basic determinants of mobility. Her conclusions also fly in the face of findings by Kohen et al. (1977), which suggest that advancement is more likely to occur among individuals who change employers than those who do not.

Actually, the results of these studies may not be as disparate as they appear at first glance. There are differences in definitions of occupation in the various studies, as well as differences in method, which account for the findings. Of most significance is the fact that Freedman (1969) used firms as her sampling base rather than individuals. Her sample was made up of entrants into defined firms and she examined the progress of men within these firms. As is clear from her data, most of her sample had labor market experience (78%) before entering the studied establishments. Although the hiring practices of these firms are not described in detail, it would appear that they did not hire new entrants to any great extent.

The available research results suggest that several things occur during the work establishment period that influence the eventual careers of individuals. One major function of work establishment is that of "correcting errors" (Ornstein, 1976). The acceptance of an initial job offer is the product of at least two decision processes: one related to occupational choice and one related to the evaluation and acceptance of the job offer. Errors can occur in either or both of these. The Kohen et al. (1977) data on job separations indicate that dissatisfaction with the work, conditions, location, and pay accounts for over one-third of all voluntary separations from jobs. Employment can quickly reveal to the individual errors in prior decision processes.

A second function of work establishment is to reduce discrepancies between expectations and reality. It appears that most people enter the labor force in positions that are beneath their status and wage expectations. Finding a better job or better wages accounted for 43% of the voluntary job separations reported by Kohen et al. (1977). All studies generally find that whether an individual changes employers or stays within an internal labor market, there is a steady increase in wages during the period of work establishment. Ornstein (1976) suggests that increased wages are the primary determinant in the decision to change jobs, although Freedman (1969) indicates that the realistic anticipation of higher future wages is a major factor in the decision to remain with a particular establishment.

A third function of work establishment is introducing the worker to the volatility of the labor market. The odds are better than one in three that entry-level workers will lose their employment involuntarily. Even though voluntary job-changing is the best way to secure occupational mobility, workers have to be able to deal with nonvoluntary separations in a positive manner.

The fourth, perhaps most important, function of work establishment is that of linking a worker with an establishment or organization that has an internal labor market. At some point in the process, as Freedman (1969) has indicated, occupational mobility becomes dependent upon establishing attachments to a stable organization that provides security against layoffs (or a cushion if they occur), adequate wages, and future prospects for both wage increases and promotions. The literature on vocational choice and career development tends to emphasize occupations to the exclusion of the organizations in which occupations are found. Freedman's (1969) research, in conjunction with that of Ornstein (1976), suggests that work establishment involves *both* finding an occupation compatible with interests, needs, and abilities, and finding an organization that provides for relatively permanent exercise of these traits.

Intervention in Work Establishment

We have indicated that work establishment is a much-neglected aspect of the career development process. Consequently, there is a dearth of specific, empirically based intervention strategies and techniques to deal with it. There are, however, some general considerations and approaches for dealing with work establishment problems which may be encountered by persons with disabilities.

It is basic to consider any potential placement in relation to the prior work establishment history and career pattern of the individual. Persons who have developmental disabilities, or who acquire their disabilities in adolescence or early adulthood before any clear work establishment process has occurred, will probably run the greatest risk during the process of work establishment. Essentially these individuals have no prior ties to the work force, organizations, or occupations, and may need special assistance when entering a new job.

Among individuals who attained establishment before the onset of disability, the least risk is encountered among those who can return to their same occupation with their previous employers (Jaffe, Day, and Adams, 1964). The next lowest risks are individuals who return to work in the same occupation with a different employer, followed by those who return to a different occupation with the same firms, and those who return to a different occupation with a different firm (Jaffe et al., 1964). In other words, the greater the similarity between the occupation and employer of the first job obtained after rehabilitation to that of the occupation and employer before disability, the more likely that the individual will be able to pick up the threads of pre-disability work establishment and career development processes and resume a "normal" developmental path. Information gathered during the initial efforts to place the individual, as well as that gathered during the period of adjustment to the original placement, provides a valuable baseline assessment of problems that may be encountered in work establishment and provides for finding effective means of overcoming these problems.

The effort required to secure the original placement of the individual indicates the individual's potential ability to independently change positions or employers. The individual who requires extensive selective placement assistance, coupled with job restructuring and modification services, is likely to need the same kind of assistance in making the transitions necessary for work establishment. Even in situations where an initial, tentative attachment to an organization has been achieved, it may be necessary to work with supervision and management to assure that normal establishment and promotional channels are open. Job and environmental restructuring beyond the immediate "rehabilitation" placement may be needed. These needs may be met at the time the original placement is made by close work with management and supervision. However, provisions must be made to meet these needs even if they arise later.

Similarly, the problems encountered during the initial work adjustment as well as the relative success of techniques used to resolve them provide an indication of potential service needs *after* the individual has made a job change during work establishment. It was indicated earlier that *each* change requires a new work adjustment, the magnitude of which may be roughly related to the degree of the change. An organizational promotion from clerk-typist I to clerk-typist II may involve only a minor change in job duties and responsibilities, with the individual remaining at the same work station, surrounded by the same co-workers. At the other extreme, a work establishment job change could be as potentially traumatic as the initial placement itself and involve a new employer, new work rules, new co-workers, new job duties, and so on.

The same types of services as were outlined earlier under work adjustment may be necessary.

An insidious, easily overlooked, aspect of work establishment involves the increased familial, social, and community roles and responsibilities that come about as a natural consequence of being reintegrated into the labor force. Disability benefits, welfare payments, and entry-level wages provide for a meager existence, but one that is relatively free of many responsibilities. The increased wage levels that occur during work establishment provide the individual with discretionary funds to be spent on things other than basic necessities. Increased occupational levels carry with them social status and prestige which has to be recognized. Social obligations and expectations develop through work group memberships. All of these stem directly from stable participation in the work force. A strictly work-oriented approach may neglect these matters, which Krantz (1970) has called the "critical employment-coupled behaviors." They are critical in the sense that unless the individual can cope with and adapt to changes in other spheres of life activity, problems in maintaining employment will arise.

THE CAREER ENHANCEMENT
PHASE OF CAREER DEVELOPMENT

We have defined *career enhancement* as a broad process that subsumes work adjustment and work establishment. The latter are microprocesses within the total set of coping, adapting, planning, and risk-taking activities characterizing career development.

Although a great deal has been written on the subject of "career development," this literature focuses almost totally on making initial career and occupational choices. The issue of what happens to people after they make these choices has not received much attention. There is some research in progress, such as the career pattern study being undertaken by Super and his associates, that may produce necessary information on the career development of persons in general to serve as a baseline for discussing the patterns of people with disabilities.

The area of adult development, which includes the vital areas of career and vocation, has been very much neglected. Only in the past few years have psychologists broken out of developmental models that presume that development is completed in childhood or adolescence. Researchers have begun to look to adult development for its own sake. Levinson et al. (1978) have recently reported the results of an intensive study of adult male development.

Levinson et al. identified three discrete periods or "eras" that characterize the development of the adult male: early adult, middle adult, and late adult. These eras are joined by three major transition periods: early adult, occurring between 17 and 22 years of age; mid-life, occurring between 40 and 45; and late adult, occurring between 60 and 65. There are numerous qualitative differences among ways of life in each of the three major eras, with the transitions occurring at the times these changes occur.

Of particular interest and relevance is Levinson's point that most males "undergo a mid-life change in style of work and living" which is at least in part occasioned by physical factors. As Levinson et al. (1978) put it:

> Although biological decline ordinarily occurs gradually, several small changes often bring about a major qualitative drop in body function by the early forties. This change may require considerable accommodation in the man's style of living and social roles, especially with regard to work (p. 25).

The most obvious examples are individuals who engage in strenuous physical occupations such as laboring and professional athletics. There are numerous other occupations, not so obvious, in which the same thing occurs. For example, major scientific discoveries are usually made by young persons (Kuhn, 1970), and, by mid-life, scientists commonly turn to teaching or administrative occupations, rather than continue creative research work. This could happen because body functions have changed.

The career ladders and lattices associated with specific occupations can interact with the kinds of physical and psychological factors mentioned above to increase the probability of change. The career ladders for many occupations are relatively short, enabling the individual to reach the top of the ladder by the late 30s. Organizational career ladders tend to be pyramids, with advancement being increasingly competitive or restricted. Persons in their 30s who have reached an initial supervisory level position may find further advancement blocked in a youthful organization if administrators and managers are in their 40s. It could be 15 to 20 years before death and retirement create new advancement possibilities.

Occupational and organization career lattices may allow for movement into related occupations and facilitate transition and change. For the most part, however, workers are confronted with the choice between continuing in an occupation or making a major occupational change.

The available research evidence suggests that most people decide to continue with what they are doing. Levinson et al. (1978) indicate that recognizing that one's early career goals will not be achieved is an ingredient in the mid-life transition. Part of the transition involves adjusting to this fact and making the necessary adaptations in vocational goals, values, and plans. Studies of the career patterns of specific occupational groups, such as machinists and assembly line workers, show this same general pattern of secure, steady employment (Crites, 1969). At the same time, it should be recognized that this cultural pattern may not persist. The concept of mid-life career change has gained a fair degree of social acceptability in the past few years. A recent special issue of the *Vocational Guidance Quarterly* (Hitchcock, 1977) was devoted exclusively to the subject. The next decade may show an increase in the number of persons who decide not to continue in an occupation and to make a major mid-life career change instead. This can be an exceptionally stressful time and may require individuals to engage in training to acquire new occupational knowledge and skills before reestablishing themselves in the work force in a new occupation.

The available research literature on career patterns shows that they are remarkably flat. Most workers tend to remain at the same occupational level throughout their entire working lives (Crites, 1969). This is in distinct contrast to the common theoretical view of career development, which tends to focus upon steady advancement to progressively higher occupational levels. The Horatio Alger, stockboy to company president approach to career development is not supported by empirical evidence.

Levinson et al.'s (1978) formulation of adult development may provide the source for a more accurate view of career development by contrasting the qualities of early adulthood with those of mid-life:

> Early adulthood produces qualities of strength, quickness, endurance, and output. Middle adulthood is a season when other qualities can ripen: wisdom, judiciousness, magnanimity, unsentimental compassion, breadth of perspective, the tragic sense (p. 25).

The period of work establishment may, for most workers, also be the period of advancement and Horatio Algerism. Career development beyond that point may be more closely tied to personal growth and development than to occupational growth. It seems most likely that this reevaluation is similar to that which occurs in adaptation to disability (Wright, 1960), when individuals can take a deeper look at themselves in relation to their work and come to value what they have rather than what they do not have or cannot attain. This implies that career development involves a deepening of personal and work values. This can enable individuals to derive more satisfaction from work and find a heightened sense of vocational identity which could help them to accept maintaining themselves in particular occupations. This would involve a coping and adapting process (Shontz, 1975), even to the extent of experiencing crisis and resolution (Kroll et al., 1970).

Intervention in Long-Range Career Enhancement

The one certainty in career development is that the individual will encounter some type of mid-life or mid-career crisis. "Having a crisis at this time is not in itself pathological. Indeed, the person who goes through this period with minimal discomfort may be denying that his life must change, for better or worse. He is thus losing an opportunity for personal development" (Levinson et al., 1978, p. 26). The obvious intervention approach is to assist the individual to deal with this crisis. Doing so involves the use of a number of techniques related to anxiety reduction and management, development of coping skills, and so on. Not to be neglected are the approaches for dealing with career crisis described by Kroll et al. (1970).

Entine (1977) has pointed out that mid-career counseling includes both personal and career counseling. Personal counseling includes elements that assist the individual to understand the nature of the changes that are being experienced and to deal effectively with these changes. This assistance may include such things as value clarification. Career counseling includes elements that help the individual understand the available career and occupational options and how to deal with them. Super (1977) has noted that experienced adults have a different set of options than adolescents or young adults. Some options are closed because of age, physical, or preparation time factors. Other options, however, only become available to individuals with certain kinds of prior experiences. These have to be made known to the individual. It might be noted, in passing, that this requires different sets of occupational information materials than those now available and used for career counseling of adolescents and young adults.

The third broad intervention strategy in career development deals directly with the career change issue. For some individuals, a career change will be an integral part of career development. This can require counseling for decision-making and choice, training and vocational preparation, placement, and a gamut of post-placement services.

A fourth intervention strategy has to be available to deal with problems associated with withdrawal from the labor force. At some point in time, withdrawal is necessary, whether it is the result of the cumulative effects of disability or simply retirement. Activity and leisure counseling approaches (Entine, 1977; McDaniels, 1977) are of importance here, as are the personal counseling and crisis intervention approaches mentioned previously.

IMPLICATIONS FOR REHABILITATION SERVICES

The time during which work adjustment, work establishment, and ongoing career enhancement typically occur have major implications for the provision of post-placement services in vocational rehabilitation. It probably takes about 1 year before initial work adjustment is stabilized. A variety of problems may occcur during this period and may have to be dealt with. The research evidence suggests that needed assistance is either not being provided to large numbers of persons or not being provided for long periods of time after placement. Zadny and James (1976) reported that only 12% of Alaska VR clients were kept in Status 22—In employment for 9 months or more during fiscal year 1975 (FY 75). Similarly, the national figures for FY 75 indicate that post-employment services are typically provided to less than 10% of the clients served by the state-federal VR program.

It has also been noted that the reestablishment of a person with a disability in the work force probably takes about 5 years to achieve. During this period, two or more job changes typically occur that may require placement and work adjustment services. The extent to which these services are provided, or even the extent to which they are needed, is not known. There are barriers to the provision of work establishment services. The lack of awareness among rehabilitation counselors and others of the concept of work establishment is one significant barrier. Counselors are simply not oriented to thinking in terms of a 5-year post-placement obligation, nor are agencies well equipped to actually provide services over 5 years. Record retention policies calling for the disposal of records 3 years after closure can be a major barrier to long-term follow up. A policy designed to protect all people from the misuse of outdated information has the long-run effect of preventing some persons with disabilities from receiving needed services.

Similar barriers to the provision of needed career enhancement services exist. A person may encounter a mid-life career crisis and be unable to receive needed services because prior rehabilitation services have removed the individual's vocational limitation. It may be that the kinds of long-run, post-placement services that have been discussed in this chapter could best be provided by private rehabilitation programs rather than the state-federal VR program. Private programs could provide needed assistance without going through the legislative and regulatory rigamarole inherent in the state-federal program.

The empirical knowledge necessary for planning and developing post-placement services is lacking. It is not known what happens to persons with disabilities in the long run. Studies such as those that have been conducted with workers in general in the areas of work adjustment, work establishment, and career enhancement are desperately needed. These studies could be conducted at rather low cost. Replication of existing designs, methods, and analyses could produce valuable information. The knowledge barrier is one that is easiest to attack at this point in time and the one that, if eliminated, could have real impact on the provision of post-placement services. It is the barrier that should receive priority attention.

REFERENCES

Azrin, N., Flores, T., and Kaplan, S. 1975. Job finding club: A group assisted program for obtaining employment. Behav. Res. Ther. 13:17–27.

Bandura, A. 1969. Principles of Behavior Modification. Holt, Rinehart & Winston, Inc., New York.

Bandura, A. 1971. Psychological Modeling. Aldine-Atherton, Chicago.

Bandura, A. 1977. Social Learning Theory. Prentice-Hall, Inc., Englewood Cliffs, New Jersey.

Bernstein, D. 1976. Anxiety management. In W. Craighead, A. Kazdin, and H. Mahoney (eds.), Behavior Modification: Principles, Issues, and Applications, pp. 183–199. Houghton Mifflin Co., Boston.

Braude, L. 1975. Work and Workers. Praeger Publishers, New York.

Burke, F., Weir, T., and Duncan, G. 1976. Informal helping relationships in work organizations. Acad. Manage. J. 19:370–377.

Crites, J. 1969. Vocational Psychology. McGraw-Hill Book Co., New York.

Dawis, R. 1976. The Minnesota Theory of Work Adjustment. In B. Bolton (ed.), Handbook of Measurement and Evaluation in Rehabilitation, pp. 227–248. University Park Press, Baltimore.

Dawis, R., and Lofquist, L. 1976. Personality style and the process of work adjustment. J. Counsel. Psychol. 23:55–59.

Entine, A. 1977. Counseling for mid-life and beyond. Voc. Guid. Quart. 25:332–336.

Freedman, M. 1969. The Process of Work Establishment. Columbia University Press, New York.

French, J., Rodgers, W., and Cobb, S. 1974. Adjustment as person-environment fit. In G. Coelho, D. Hamburg, and J. Adams (eds.), Coping and Adaptation, pp. 316–333. Basic Books, Inc., New York.

Goldfried, M., and Davison, G. 1976. Clinical Behavior Therapy. Holt, Rinehart & Winston, New York.

Hershenson, D. 1974. Vocational guidance and the handicapped. In E. Herr (ed.), Vocational Guidance and Human Development, pp. 478–501. Houghton Mifflin Co., Boston.

Hitchcock, A. 1977. Guest editor's introduction. Voc. Guid. Quart. 25:292–293.

Jaffe, A., Day, L., and Adams, W. 1964. Disabled Workers in the Labor Market. Bedminister Press, Totawa, New Jersey.

Karen, R. 1974. An Introduction to Behavior Theory and Its Applications. Harper & Row Publishers, New York.

Kohen, A., Grasso, J., Myers, S., and Shields, P. 1977. Career Thresholds Volume 6: A Longitudinal Study of the Educational and Labor Market Experience of Young Men. Government Printing Office, Washington, D.C.

Korman, A. 1970. Toward an hypothesis of work behavior. J. Appl. Psychol. 54:31–41.

Korman, A. 1971. Industrial and Organizational Psychology. Prentice-Hall, Inc., Englewood Cliffs, New Jersey.

Krantz, G. 1970. Critical vocational behaviors. J. Rehab. 37(4):14–16.

Kroll, A., Dinklage, L., Lee, J., Morley, E., and Wilson, E. 1970. Career Development: Growth and Crisis. John Wiley & Sons, Inc., New York.

Kuhn, T. 1970. The Structure of Scientific Revolutions. 2nd Ed. The University of Chicago Press, Chicago.

Levinson, D., Darrow, C., Klein, E., Levinson, M., and McKee, B. 1978. The Seasons of a Man's Life. Alfred A. Knopf, Inc., New York.

Lofquist, L., and Dawis, R. 1969. Adjustment To Work: A Psychological View of Man's Problems in a Work Oriented Society. Appleton-Century-Crofts, New York.

McDaniels, C. 1977. Leisure and career development at mid-life: A rationale. Voc. Guid. Quart. 25:344-350.

Meichenbaum, D. 1977. Cognitive Behavior Modification, Plenum Publishing Corp., New York.

Moos, R., and Tsu, V. 1977. The crisis of physical illness: An overview. In R. Moos (ed.), Coping with Physical Illness, pp. 3-21. Plenum Publishing Corp., New York.

Ornstein, M. 1976. Entry into the American Labor Force. Academic Press, Inc., New York.

Parnes, H., Jusenius, D., Blau, F., Nestel, G., Shortlidge, R., and Sandell, S. 1976. Dual Careers Volume 4: A Longitudinal Analysis of the Labor Market Experience of Women. Government Printing Office, Washington, D.C.

Roethlisberger, F., and Dickson, W. 1940. Management and the Worker. Harvard University Press, Cambridge, Massachusetts.

Rose, S. 1977. Group Therapy: A Behavioral Approach. Prentice-Hall, Inc., Englewood Cliffs, New Jersey.

Roy, D. 1952. Quota restriction and goldbricking in a machine shop. Am. J. Sociol. 57:427-442.

Roy, D. 1960. "Banana time." Job Satisfaction and informal interaction. Hum. Organ. 18:158-168.

Shontz, F. 1975. The Psychological Aspects of Physical Illness and Disability. Macmillan Publishing Co., Inc., New York.

Slocum, W. 1966. Occupational Careers. Aldine Publishing Co., Chicago.

Staats, A., and Staats, C., 1963. Complex Human Behavior. Holt, Rinehart, & Winston, Inc., New York.

Stuart, R. 1977. Self-help group approach to self-management. In R. Stuart (ed.), Behavioral Self-Management: Strategies, Techniques, and Outcomes. Brunner/Mazel, New York.

Super, D. 1957. The Psychology of Careers. Harper & Row Publishers, New York.

Super, D. 1977. Vocational maturity in mid-career. Voc. Guid. Quart. 25:294-302.

Tolbert, E. 1974. Counseling For Career Development. Houghton Mifflin Co., Boston.

Vandergoot, D., Jacobsen, R., and Worrall, J. 1977. New directions for placement-related and practical research in the rehabilitation process: A strategy paper. Project PREP, Human Resources Center, Albertson, New York.

Wright, B. 1960, Physical Disability: A Psychological Approach. Harper & Row Publishers, New York.

Zadny, J., and James, L. 1976. Another View on Placement: State of the Art 1976. Regional Rehabilitation Research Institute, Portland State University, Portland, Oregon.

Chapter 10

Linking
Vocational Rehabilitation
and the World of Work
The Business and
Industry Advisory Council

Carl Puleo

Editors's note: This chapter provides an example of how to use organizations to make local labor markets function more efficiently. This increased efficiency is generated by, among other things, increased quantity and quality of local labor market information. It also can be fostered by tailoring training and job preparation to the local labor market. Although the Business Industry Advisory Council is basically a formal framework for the transmission of labor market information, it can evolve into an effective, informal mechanism that can benefit rehabilitants, counselors, and employers. The Council also offers employers an opportunity to lower their hiring and training costs when the costs of training can be shifted from the employer to a public program.

The success of advisory councils is not automatic. The use of a council can offer the rehabilitation professional a source of lifetime contacts in the business community, but care must be taken to ensure that a council does not degenerate into a figurehead without a real role in the rehabilitation program. Therefore, when initiating and developing an advisory council, it is important to specify its role within the program and to make clear the kind of relationship desired.

Advisory councils represent an approach that rehabilitation may take in defining a truly cooperative relationship with the employing community. Thompson and McEwen (1958)[1] suggest that an organization may deal either competitively or cooperatively with the environment. Three types of cooperative strategy are noted: bargaining, co-optation, and coalition. Bargaining is an attempt to formalize the structure of competition in order to give it greater stability. This approach reflects attempts on the part of rehabilitation agencies to ensure full considerations of their clients by employers, who are encouraged to look more carefully at these workers than they otherwise might. Placement and job development efforts give job-seekers an edge that they might not otherwise have.

Co-optation is a formalized means of ensuring ongoing communication between organizations. This increases the likelihood that they will find compatible

---

[1] Thompson, J. D., and McEwen, W. J. 1958. Organizational goals environment: Goal setting as an interaction process. Am Sociol. Rev. 23:23–31.

goals. Advisory councils with a standing membership that meets periodically can be seen as examples of co-optation. "Co-optation is more than expediency. By giving a potential supporter a position of power and often of responsibility in the organization, the organization gains his awareness and understanding of the problems it faces."[1]

Throughout the service process, the rehabilitation agency can gain knowledge and awareness through a relationship with the employing community. Employers' needs, including a need for qualified workers, may be met as well. This process is not automatic, however, and mutually satisfactory structure for interaction must be created.

The third form of cooperative strategy, coalition, represents a situation in which two or more organizations form close bonds to achieve a common purpose. This approach is less common due to the potential threat posed to the separate integrity of the organizations.

The most significant objective of the vocational rehabilitation process, and one that is not always accomplished, is effectively placing people with disabilities in meaningful jobs in the business and industrial communities of our country. Effective placement has always been a challenge to vocational rehabilitation professionals, and it continues to be a challenge today. One of the basic obstacles to effective placement has been the inability of rehabilitation professionals to recognize the need to integrate rehabilitation practice with its ultimate goal, the appropriate job for a person with a disability. Some rehabilitation professionals, because of their training and very possibly because of the personal attributes that led them to a helping profession, are equipped to work effectively and comfortably in carrying out the process of vocational rehabilitation with clients in the various rehabilitation and workshop settings. However, some professional rehabilitation training programs have insufficiently stressed the development of skills necessary to find jobs for clients with work disabilities.

CLASSICAL APPROACH TO THE PLACEMENT PROCESS

Historically, the ultimate step in the rehabilitation process, the placement of the trained person into competitive employment, has been shared by both the state vocational counselor and the rehabilitation or education facility in which the person's rehabilitation took place. Often there was not a clear-cut commitment to placement and this resulted in a delay in placement or in inappropriate placement.

Many rehabilitation facilities and workshops, often claiming insufficient funding, only maintained the responsibility for vocational rehabilitation up to the point of discharge. Hence, the burden of responsibility for placement reverted to the vocational counselor. Because of heavy case load demands, coupled with the unique and time-consuming problem of job development in the placement process, counselors often found it necessary to rely heavily on their clientele to develop their own jobs with little direct intervention and assistance.

The classical approach taken by rehabilitation facilities and workshops was to move persons through their vocational programs. The programs included work experience training and skill training centered around the specific types of subcontract work performed by the facility, usually some type of assembly or light branch work. Whether these skills were specifically related to jobs in the community was often not considered. Very likely, facility staff relied heavily upon the concept of transferable skills as a substitute for considering what the labor market demand actually was.

Consequently, the following scenario seems to be the standard approach to the placement of a person with a disability:

A. The person is referred to a rehabilitation facility by a vocational counselor after disability and eligibility criteria are established by the referring agency.

B. Upon receipt of referral information, including pertinent medical, psychological, and psychiatric data; precautions; and other specific factors that might limit vocational objectives, an intake interview is scheduled. During this interview, pertinent history is obtained, the facility's vocational program is described, and a tour of the facility is conducted. The person is also seen by the facility's medical director, who reviews the individual's medical history and needs.

C. A preadmission conference is held to determine whether the individual can be appropriately served by the facility. This conference includes the social worker, medical director, supervisor of vocational evaluation, referring counselor, and other facility staff. At this conference, a tentative plan is developed for the individual including: 1) selection and scheduling of evaluation techniques, 2) special evaluation services; e.g., physical capacities evaluation, and 3) assignment to a facility evaluator who will be responsible for individual programming and reporting.

D. The evaluation process reveals the options open for further vocational rehabilitation; i.e., work adjustment training, specific skill training, and job-seeking skills training.

E. Once the individuals are considered "work ready," they are referred back to the vocational counselor for placement. This placement process is often a responsibility shared by the state vocational counselor and a placement counselor from the facility.

F. At this point, the task is to convince an employer that this individual with a disability should be hired, since the primary responsibility of vocational rehabilitation has been dispatched by the rehabilitation specialists. Now the burden is shifted to the employer who is entreated to fulfill a social responsibility, by hiring a rehabilitated individual.

A very basic and important issue is frequently missing from this scenario: more intentional involvement of the business and industrial community with the whole rehabilitation process.

Historically, the rehabilitation community appeared to adopt the attitude that they, the experts, would provide whatever rehabilitation seemed appropriate and necessary for individuals up to a point where competitive employment was possible. Then it was up to the business community to take these "trained handicapped" persons and put them to work.

However, in the past few years, and basically as a result of a federally sponsored program called "Projects with Industry" (PWI), there has been a significant shift in the relationship of the business community with the rehabilitation community and it is beginning to have a remarkable impact upon the whole concept of vocational rehabilitation. This impact is the closing of the gap between the employer and the rehabilitation agency.

The Rehabilitation Act of 1973 and resulting regulations strengthened the nation's vocational rehabilitation services in several ways. One serious gap closed because of the development of the Projects with Industry (PWI) program. The gap in rehabilitation services that Congress perceived was an undue separation between employers and the rehabilitation community. The law authorized the Department of Health, Education and Welfare (HEW) to "make contracts or jointly financed cooperative arrangements with employers and rehabilitation organizations for projects designed to prepare individuals with disabilities for gainful and suitable employment in a realistic work setting and such other services as may be necessary for such individuals to continue to engage in such employment."

The intent of this legislation was to facilitate the entry of persons with severe disabilities into realistic work settings and to encourage greater participation in rehabilitating such individuals by private employers. It was to meet these needs that the Projects with Industry concept evolved. The Business Advisory Council was set up to ensure successful placement of these trained persons in meaningful jobs. These councils have created a partnership concept that works.

BUSINESS AND REHAB: NEW PARTNERS

The basic shift in the vocational rehabilitation process from what was previously described as the historical or classical approach is a change in attitude and practice on the part of rehabilitation specialists. More counselors are now seeking guidance and support from business and union leadership so that rehabilitation facilities can provide services and training to suit the labor demand of the locality. This means that the business community is up front in the process—business becomes a partner in the rehabilitation process. Before, employers were passive recipients of job applicants with disabilities who were referred by the rehabilitation community.

The Business Advisory Council is the key to this partnership. Although this council can take on different forms in different communities, it is instructive first to consider a general advisory council structure, and, second, to look at a specific business advisory council program that has had a relative degree of success.

Advisory Council

A significant function of the PWI program is focusing rehabilitation activity on specific needs of business and industry, rather than relying on the chance that an appropriate job will turn up when an individual completes some arbitrary training program that may or may not be responsive to the skill needs currently being demanded by business or industry. With a PWI focus, the indiviudal's aptitudes and skills are evaluated against the standards of performance established by the specific industry as a qualification for employment. This focus imposes a need for communication between business and industry and the rehabilitation community in order to translate job descriptions and skill needs into rehabilitation training objectives and evaluation criteria.

The Advisory Council is a working group composed of representatives of businesses and industries in a given geographical area. The members should be aware of the employment outlook for the businesses that they represent. An important objective of the Advisory Council is to provide sound advice to the project director of PWI and hence to the rehabilitation facility. Issues that the Advisory Council address include:

Skill requirements and standards of performance for jobs in identified
    employment areas
Specific job requirements in selected career paths
Selection criteria for trainees
Training curricula, media of instruction, work and personal adjustment,
    follow-along service, and feedback to the training program.
Placement assistance and support
Development of project plans and definition of benchmarks for measure-
    ment of progress

An additional reason for convening an advisory council is establishing a cooperative link and shared responsibility between business and the rehabilitation facility with the idea of finding jobs for trained workers who happen to have disabilities. This cooperative relationship could help the business community in a number of ways. It would be one way to identify a source of competent employees. It could serve to open up the opportunity for qualified rehabilitation specialists to provide job retention counseling services to companies that have a high turnover. The relationship also provides a valuable tool for business because prospective employees would be trained to perform skills relevant to business while allowing business to evaluate prospective employees before placing them on the payroll. This also helps businesses to satisfy their Affirmative Action compliance requirements.

Other areas of concern include recruitment of additional council members and establishment of additional training/placement sites in response to surveys of labor market needs. It is obvious that the Advisory Council can participate actively in the rehabilitation process.

Advisory councils have been organized around areas where their impact is most beneficial: training, business readiness, and placement. Subcommittees of the advisory council typically provide leadership assistance and guidance in such areas as:

Defining skills and abilities that a trained individual from a program should possess
Developing the curriculum to produce the skills and abilities
Acquainting the trainee with the business environment
Participating in the course instruction where appropriate
Obtaining placements for individuals who complete their training successfully

A given community provides a cross section of potential advisory council candidates from which to select; however, each member should have a business relationship relevant to the situation of people with disabilities. Members should be able to provide expert counsel in the process of vocational rehabiliation, primarily with reference to the appropriate jobs available. Such an Advisory Council might meet monthly with subcommittee meetings as needed.

Business Advisory Council—The New Haven Model

The New Haven model of of a Business Advisory Council can now be examined more specifically. The Easter Seal Goodwill Industries Rehabilitation Center of New Haven has accepted the responsibility and challenge of working in cooperation with the employer community to develop programs that will change attitudes and patterns of training, hiring, retention, and advancement of qualified workers who have disabilities. The intention of the participants in the New Haven program is to obtain suitable training and/or job slots in business and industry for people with work disabilities. In addition, the process is an attempt to develop an understanding and awareness on the part of industry regarding people with disabilities, contributing to the achievement of their ultimate goal of increased assimilation into competitive jobs.

This is accomplished through a combination of four distinct methods. The first involves continuous communication with area industries and businesses. Second, industries and businesses choosing to participate in the project through training and/or placement of three or more agency rehabilitants are encouraged to assign a liaison person to work with the project staff in identifying suitable job slots. The liaison person can provide job coaching and help make the transition from rehabilitation center to actual competitive employment as successful as possible. The third method is to closely follow up the placement with in-plant liaison people for at least 1 year after the placement is made. The project staff also works with the new employee's supervisor and even co-workers during this follow-up phase, since job success often depends upon the new worker's acceptance by co-workers and front-line supervisors. It is essential that the rehabilitant receive strong support, especially during the initial phase of employment, from the project staff, the liaison, and/or the supervisor. The fourth method is to invite participating industries and businesses to the Rehabilitation Center for orientation meetings. Frequently, these meetings include representatives of top management, personnel, and production. These people can discuss important issues with the project staff, such as the progress of the project. They can provide valuable information regarding innovative ideas, methods to increase the number of persons placed in industry, and can act as consultants to the Center on matters such as employment of persons with disabilities, personnel policies, or workers' compensation. This business and industrial support both resulted in the formation of and is the result of the Business Advisory Council, which is the supporting resource for the PWI program.

The New Haven Advisory Council is composed of leading representatives from business and industry, civic and nonprofit organizations, state rehabilitation agencies, educational institutions, rehabilitation consumers, and others. The Advisory Council's charge is to identify ways and means by which business and industry can establish meaningful policies and procedures that will encourage the training and employment, retention, and advancement of trained rehabilitants in the competitive labor market. The Council also provides a liaison between the professional rehabilitation community and the employers' establishments and rleated organizations such as unions. It provides a vehicle for keeping employers apprised of the availability of skilled people who have disabilities, serves as a spokesman for employers in relating to the rehabilitation community, identifies and establishes priority areas of training and employment, and encourages employers to provide leadership and assume greater fiscal and technical responsibility for rehabilitation programs. In addition, the council participates in the development of long-range plans, including legislative enactments, and provides advice and guidance in ways of using the mass media to promote the training and employment of persons with disabilities.

In the New Haven model, the chairman of the Advisory Council is always elected from the business community. At no time will the Council, or any subcommittee of the Council, for that matter, be chaired by a rehabilitation professional from the Rehabilitation Center. There is a strong feeling on the part of both the facility staff and the business and industrial volunteer leadership that, in order to maintain the integrity and strength of the Advisory Council and its subcommittee system, the chairperson must be a business representative. This Council is staffed by the project director for PWI and other PWI staff as needed.

Committees

Presently, the Advisory Council has 25 members from the business community and meets quarterly to receive reports from its active committees, which are the working arms of the Council. There are seven committees addressing specific training areas:

Data Processing	Food Service
Office Practice	Manufacturing
Custodial	Teller Training
Retail Sales	

Another committee addressing a specific need is the Job-Seeking Skills Advisory Committee. This committee deals with both the problems of job-seeking skills and job retention.

The committees address, among other things, the development of a curriculum tailored to meet business standards and requirements that will help a successful trainee be "work prepared." Thus, the curriculum addresses the needs of the business community in which the trainee will most likely be placed.

The committees have also taken on the task of securing from the business community whatever equipment is needed to provide the appropriate specific training.

These committees represent over 80 different businesses in the local market area. They consist of both Advisory Council members and other business representatives not on the Council. The committees have the option of separating into subcommittee structure for the purpose of dividing work and responsibility if that seems appropriate.

The data processing committee is an example of one committee that has subdivided for practical functional purposes. This committee has four subcommittees addressing specific needs:

Technical Subcommittee Responsible for developing, refining, and reviewing course curricula and monitoring the progress of the class.

Business Subcommittee Arranges on-site visits of the class to computer installations and provides guest lectures.

Hardware/Software Subcommittee Identifies the hardware and software needed and assists in obtaining the equipment on an ongoing basis.

Placement Subcommittee Responsible for placing all graduates of the program. This subcommittee arranges interviews, job fairs, and contacts to get the trained graduate and prospective employer together. It begins its work well before the end of the course. Thus, a prospective employer can provide information to potential employees (trainees) regarding specific job techniques that can be developed before course completion.

Too much emphasis cannot be placed upon the importance of the business and industry input through the curriculum subcommittee with regard to development of a curriculum that has its roots and validity in business. The following data further amplify the importance of a business-related curriculum that cites the training performance of the New Haven-based program:

1977 Graduating Class of eight persons with severe disabilities: Seven (7) selected computer programming as a career. Average starting salary—$12,500 annually.

1978 Graduating Class of 10 persons with severe disabilities: Nine (9) selected computer programming as a career and were employed. Total annual starting salaries, $12.5 million. Average starting salary—$14,000 annually.

DEVELOPMENTAL HISTORY OF BUSINESS ADVISORY COUNCIL: THE NEW HAVEN MODEL

The recruitment of Advisory Council members was shared by the PWI project director and a recently retired IBM sales executive who also became the Council's first interim chairman. The bulk of the recruitment responsibility was given to this business person, which was a key strategy in selling the Advisory Council concept; i.e., business person selling business person. This strategy proved to be most successful in developing strength, enthusiasm, and commitment from those who have elected to become members of the Business Advisory Council.

The present Advisory Council model in place in New Haven evolved through a problem and task-oriented process. The first Advisory Council was structured to explore with the Projects with Industry staff four large identified areas of concern; namely, office practices, industrial operations, food services, and general building maintenance. The Council as a whole, approximately 80 representatives, met on a regular bimonthly basis, and the four large committees met between meetings to focus attention on work-related problems in their area of concern.

This advisory council structure and format was in place for a year and served to orient both the advisory council members with the vocational rehabilitation process and problems and the Projects with Industry staff with the needs of the business community. It did not, however, effectively serve to meet the mutual desire to isolate and attach specific problems relating to effective placement of trained, qualified workers with disabilities into jobs in the business sector.

The Advisory Council restructured itself into committee and subcommittee format, addressing specific training needs that were identified in the business community. Once the committees were restructured around a specific training need, problems were identified and responsibilities were assigned. Committees began meeting regularly to address the issues employing a results orientation, the language business people understand. The committees and subcommittees recruited additional expertise from the business community, thus expanding greatly the scope of business and industry involvement. The Advisory Council was then reduced in size to one-third, consisting primarily of chairmen of committees and subcommittees and members at large. The Advisory Council now meets quarterly, specifically to receive committee and subcommittee reports and to address problems of a more global nature.

This model has been extremely effective because the committees have established a results-oriented strategy that assigns specific responsibilities and accountabilities. It seems to ensure a dynamic posture and minimizes the risk of stagnation, without with the committee structure could be counterproductive and result in failure.

The opposite has been the case. The climate created is success oriented. It is hoped that the strategies for the relative success of the New Haven model can be sustained and improved upon.

Annual Conference

An annual function of the Business Advisory Council is an areawide, 1-day conference for business representatives and rehabilitation professionals. The thrust of the conference is to demonstrate the positive impact of the partnership between business and rehabilitation to a broad representation of the business and rehabilitation community. The conference serves as a vehicle to encourage more businesses to become involved with the vocational rehabilitation process. It also serves as a forum to acquaint business with the services available to them through the Rehabilitation Center. The center is a source of trained workers, a place for on-the-job training opportunities should a business prefer to structure its own training program, a provider of supportive counseling services to the company and to workers for job retention purposes, and a source of architectural barrier and affirmative action consultation. One strength of the annual conference is that business people can talk with other business people about jobs for trained persons with disabilities. The rehabilitation staff is a catalyst for discussion and functions as an information resource at the conference.

The Business Advisory Council and its committee and subcommittee structure in New Haven has made the difference between the historic vocational rehabilitation approach, which provides a measure of service to the client and then presents a prospective worker to an employer, and the present program of developing a real partnership between the business community and the rehabilitation community, in which both have an opportunity to gain important benefits.

Conclusion

The key to success in the New Haven model has been the strategy of having the business community play a dominant role in the planning, execution, monitoring, and evaluation of the ongoing processes of recruitment and the training and placement of workers with disabilities into meaningful jobs within the community.

The rehabilitation professionals respond to job needs and requirements that are continuously identified and monitored by the Business Advisory Committee. This response takes the form of sharpening the mechanisms of vocational rehabilitation from recruitment (outreach) through vocational evaluation, behavioral modification, work adjustment, skill training, job-seeking skills training, vocational counseling, job development, job placement, work retention counseling, and follow-up services with the worker and employer.

The Business Advisory Council gives meaningful direction to the entire vocational rehabilitation process. With this direction, rehabilitation professionals have a more practical and workable framework in which to provide vocational rehabilitation services than ever before. The challenge to the rehabilitation facility is to adapt its vocational rehabilitation process to match the real job needs and requirements of the business and industrial community, rather than following a process of rehabilitation that might ultimately have little to do with the practical needs of business.

More and more, employers are looking at their social responsibility in the community where they make profits. Social responsibility, however, must support and complement the business's primary reason for being, and that is the maximization of return on investment. The rehabilitation community must develop its programs with this in mind if the programs are to survive and keep obtaining jobs for persons with disabilities.

The Business Advisory Council concept is proving to be a model for success. The reason for success lies in the commitment to the task and objective—jobs in business and industry. This commitment to vocational rehabilitation comes about when both business and rehabilitation professionals participate in the total process from the start. When rehabilitation experts plan with attention to the requirements and needs of the business community and develop programs that address business work requirements, the partnership effort carries the process to its ultimate conclusion—meaningful jobs in business for trained persons with disabilities.

Once a facility takes the step of intentionally working in partnership with the business community in vocational rehabilitation, the process must be irreversible if credibility is to be maintained. The simple ideas that support this are: 1) the goal of vocational rehabilitation is jobs in the community, 2) jobs are in the province of the employer community—business and industry, 3) in order to develop a successful match of the worker and the job, there must be commitment to that end by both the employer and the rehabilitation community, 4) a long-lasting commitment requires active participation and involvement and 5) the job cannot be done without business and industry.

These ideas emphasize the need for a meaningful and productive cooperative relationship between business and rehabilitation. The New Haven model is a working example of a strong and binding business and rehabilitation partnership.

Chapter 11

The Role of Staff Development and Agency Administration in More Effective Job Placement

Susanne M. Bruyère

Editor's note: Staff training and development are essential to any successful organization, even as they can be crucial in career development. Dr. Bruyère considers the role of staff development and agency administration from an organizational point of view. This method can be applied to any agency program or facility that provides rehabilitation services.

Dr. Bruyère points out that there must be a needs assessment for placement training. Not every counselor must be trained in all areas of placement. For trainers to teach placement skills, not only must they know the skill levels of counselors, but also they must know how placement happens, i.e., what tasks lead to successful placements. She maintains that more research must be conducted before these tasks can be isolated.

Placement training should be systematic. Such training is best cast within the organization as a whole. Doing so would enable trainers to develop optimum placement curricula and help trainees to be prepared to practice what they have learned. As placement occurs in this organizational support system, Dr. Bruyère suggests that continuing education will play a major role in the transmission and maintenance of placement skills.

The chapter also considers incentives. If counselors are to perform in certain ways, not only must the performance standards be made clear, but also they should be rewarded for success. The rehabilitation system has a set of incentives, albeit implicit, that does reward certain behavior. If, for example, counselors are to be evaluated according simply to the number of placements they make, they may respond with placements of low quality. If, on the other hand, counselors are to be evaluated according to the quality and quantity of placements they make, more attention may be given to high-quality placements. Changing evaluation criteria may call for weighted case closure, as well as giving priority for service delivery to persons with severe disabilities.

This chapter offers an overview of ways in which an agency placement effort can be made more effective through the joint efforts of both staff development personnel and agency administration. Training is increasingly used by both public and private organizations not only to remediate employee performance deficits, but to deal with a variety of internal and external problems and opportunities in a manner that contributes to the achievement of overall organizational objectives. Too often, however, failure of training to make marked improvements in organizational change or in employee performance is inappropriately attributed to an inadequacy in the knowledge, skill, or enthusiasm of the trainer or the ability and motivation of the trainee. Seldom is sufficient attention paid to the mutual responsibility that staff development and agency administration share to assure that organizational and performance changes occur.

Today job placement training is receiving new emphasis in vocational rehabilitation because of the heightened trend toward accountability and the need for periodic updating of skills through continuing education. A growing number of special interest groups with vocal and able advocates are competing for limited resources to start or sustain their efforts. As a result, existing human service programs, such as vocational rehabilitation, must provide concrete proof of their effectiveness to justify their continuation. Increasing stress upon accountability has taken the form of compiling statistics indicating successful closure and job placement rates as indicators of the effectiveness of the vocational rehabilitation (VR) program. In addition, the recent emphasis to serve the more severe disabilities requires that placement efforts be closely scrutinized to assure that rehabilitation approaches to placement are the most effective for this population.

In response to this heightened need for effective approaches to job placement, many rehabilitation agencies and facilities have turned to post-employment training programs as a possible way to improve the placement performance of their personnel. Since placement, or the number of successful closures, continues to be the measure by which the value of the VR program is determined, agencies with low closure rates often look to trainers of rehabilitation personnel to teach skills that will bring about increased placement rates. However, providing placement training does not ensure that, after the trainee's return to the job, placement performance will necessarily be enhanced. The erroneous expectation of training as the sole "cure" for performance or productivity concerns often results in the frustration of agency administration, staff development personnel, and counselors.

Other chapters in this book explore specific areas of information and skills needed to more effectively place individuals with disabilities.

Identification of necessary information and skills to perform a job is a critical step in the development of professional education and training. However, as counselor educators, rehabilitation trainers, and agency administrators can verify, even the most well-conceived and comprehensive training curricula do not necessarily assure effective on-the-job performance by those who have received such training. A host of other variables, such as the specific learning needs of the individual, learner motivation, rewards in the work environment, and supporting organizational procedures, have an impact on placement performance.

The purpose of this chapter is to identify ways in which staff development personnel and agency administration can better assure that the training provided will result in more effective placement performance of rehabilitation counselors on the job. Various attempts over the past 20 years to clarify the role and function of the rehabilitation counselor are identified, and the increasing importance given to placement as an integral part of the job of the counselor is briefly discussed. The role of staff development personnel in adequately assessing training needs before the development of a training program and other considerations related to effective training are presented. Finally, management's role in creating an organizational environment that encourages placement is explored. Included are the effect of staffing patterns, clarity of placement function, rewards for effective placement efforts, and overall administrative effort in the placement process.

PLACEMENT SKILLS TRAINING: HISTORICAL PERSPECTIVE

The vocational rehabilitation (VR) system rests upon the belief that work is an important contributor to an individual's identity and sense of self-worth. Although the *degree* of emphasis may have fluctuated during the years of VR's existence, it has always been true that an important goal of rehabilitation has been the introduction or reintroduction of individuals with disabilities into the labor market. Despite this emphasis, however, the skills specifically related to job placement have only recently received attention in rehabilitation counselor education and the post-employment training of rehabilitation personnel.

In 1959, Jaques attempted to isolate the key skills needed to be a vocational rehabilitation counselor. The "critical incident" technique was applied to the work of the rehabilitation counselor to determine critical job requirements, thereby allowing more precise formulation of training needs. Jaques' study emphasized the counseling function and concluded that the skills and attitudes identified were based on psychological knowledge and an understanding of human behavior. Therefore, a psychological orientation should provide the framework for rehabilitation counselor training. No mention was specifically made of skills needed to place rehabilitated workers in jobs.

Ten years later, Muthard and Salomone (1969) studied the roles and functions of rehabilitation counselors in state agencies and private facilities, collecting basic information concerning their work tasks and traits. Results showed that the role behaviors of these counselors could be described by eight job functions; of these, affective counseling, vocational counseling, and placement duties were assigned the highest importance by the counselors surveyed. Placement was recognized as a critical function of the vocational rehabilitation counselor, although placement was reported as consuming only a small portion (7%) of the counselor's time. Most recently, efforts have been directed to more precisely specify counselor skills and skill levels. Wright and Fraser (1976) constructed an inventory of 294 job tasks of a vocational rehabilitation counselor in a state VR agency, using task analysis of VR counselor-track personnel done in the state of Wisconsin. Of these tasks, 14 were identified as being related specifically to job placement (Table 1).

Placement, in the context of vocational rehabilitation services, should not be isolated completely from the other skills needed to effectively carry out this function. The concept of placement as a part of the total rehabilitation process is a vital one; the effective vocational rehabilitation counselor must use information gathered throughout the process to aid the client in making the most appropriate vocational choice possible. However, the isolation of tasks related specifically to job placement affords the profession an opportunity to closely scrutinize areas of information and skill development that have historically been lacking in graduate training and continuing education for vocational rehabilitation counselors.

In the past, rehabilitation counselor education programs have not emphasized job placement (Scorzelli, 1975). Currently, in response to the recent interest in job placement and the identification of skills needed to better perform this part of the counselor's job, several modifications in rehabilitation counselor training have been made. A number of master's degree programs have been created that concentrate on job placement for people with disabilities. Similarly, rehabilitation counselor education programs on the graduate level have begun to add course work, often where none previously existed, to better prepare their graduates to do job placement (Usdane, 1977). As previously mentioned, to respond to the training needs of counselors already in the field, a wide variety of short-term training programs are being offered by trainers of rehabilitation personnel.

Table 1.   Job placement tasks

A.   Working with the client seeking employment
1.   Advising and directing a client in the establishment of a small business enterprise and supervising the selection and financing of business equipment.
2.   Procuring information from a client and an employer regarding the client's adjustment to a job and providing supportive counseling as necessary to ensure placement.
3.   Providing a client with employment alternatives based on resource information (e.g., D.O.T., *Occupational Briefs*, want ads).
4.   Role-playing an employment interview with a client in order to reduce anxiety and generally prepare the client for a job interview.
5.   Providing direct information to a client on an available job opening or on-the-job training program that best suits his needs and abilities.
6.   Instructing an individual or a group of clients about ways to locate job leads.
7.   Talking with a client about preparing for job interviews (e.g., appropriate dress, good grooming, positive attitudes).
8.   Providing a personal reference for a client who is seeking a job.
9.   Accompanying and assisting a client (perhaps transporting a client) to job interviews or in a job-hunting process.

B.   Developing community job opportunities
10.   Evaluating job activities in particular positions to determine if any modifications could open the positions to rehabilitation clients (e.g., safety modifications, removal of architectural barriers).
11.   Determining which (if any) industries in an assigned geographical area have paid openings or on-the-job training positions within the capabilities of clients with specific disabilities.
12.   Negotiating with an individual or organization regarding on-the-job training services for a particular client.
13.   Securing and maintaining (with clerical support) an active file on employers and training facilities.
14.   Contracting community employment resources to investigate the possibility of placing a client in gainful employment.

From *Improving Manpower Utilization: The Rehabilitation Task Performance Evaluation Scale* by G. N. Wright and R. T. Fraser, Wisconsin Studies in Vocational Rehabilitation, University of Wisconsin—Madison, Rehabilitation Research Institute, 1976. By permission.

The next section of this chapter discusses how graduate rehabilitation counselor education programs and post-employment training efforts can work together to provide rehabilitation counselors with the skills to perform more effectively in the placement role. The need for both an adequate training needs assessment of each counselor and an understanding of the organization within which the individual is going to function is explored.

THE ROLE OF TRAINING IN MORE EFFECTIVE JOB PLACEMENT

Providing Placement Training

Ideally, professional preparation and ongoing development contain an exposure to the core of information that captures the essence of the discipline and an opportunity for updating knowledge and learning new skills. Likewise, placement training for rehabilitation counselors ideally should occur as a part of the core curriculum for graduate training and be complemented by post-employment training. Graduate and undergraduate programs in rehabilitation counselor training can provide core information and techniques specifically related to job placement, such as career development theory, vocational exploration techniques, job development, job analysis and restructuring, use of labor market information in making career choices, and teaching clients job-seeking skills. With a sound, generalized background in job placement, post-employment training could provide information specifically designed to fulfill the needs of the counselor attempting to place job-ready clients in a given geographical locale. This training could include wage and hour laws, worker's compensation and insurance policies, labor union practices, and labor market trends of the state, county, or city where the trainee was located. The blending of both formal background preparation and continuing education permits potential and practicing rehabilitation counselors an opportunity to learn effective placement approaches.

Once the counselor is on the job, it is the responsibility of both agency administration and staff development personnel to enable practitioners to function effectively in their roles. Provision of continuing education is an important but not an all-inclusive way to aid counselors to more effectively accomplish their job. Even the idealized approach to job placement training just described will not necessarily ensure that the performance of graduates of rehabilitation counselor education programs, or that of practitioners who have attended short-term workshops in placement, will meet the expectations of counselor educators or agency administration. A more comprehensive and often more successful approach to staff development includes both a closer scrutiny of the needs of the individual learner and a broader perspective that keeps in focus the organizational context of the worker.

Need for Adequate Training Needs Assessment

Rehabilitation trainers and staff development personnel are being asked increasingly to assist in improving placement performance. However, all too often training is seen as a panacea for agency productivity problems, such as low placement performance, and is expected to magically alter productivity on the part of personnel. The complex array of skills needed to effectively perform the job of rehabilitation counselor makes the trainer's job of appropriately responding to the needs of the agency and the practitioner a difficult one. Training needs must be clearly defined to ensure that lack of skill in placement is actually a problem and that placement training is the answer.

Mager and Pipe (1970) provide a meaningful analogy for assessing training problems: "Solutions to training problems are like keys in locks; they don't work if they don't fit. And, if solutions aren't the right ones, the problem doesn't get solved" (p. v). Too often when there is a productivity concern in the agency, the solution chosen is training. Mager and Pipe offer a diagram that provides a concise checklist of variables that agency administrators and rehabilitation trainers might consider when analyzing performance problems (Figure 1). This approach could be useful in assessing performance problems. When applied to job placement performance, agency administrators and supervisors, staff development personnel, and the counselors themselves might ask some of these questions when assessing work performance:

1. Is it important? (Many counselors may approach placement in different ways with equal success. If placement outcome is satisfactory, it therefore may not be necessary to alter a counselor's approach to placement even if different from that of co-workers.)
2. Is the counselor aware of what is expected in the job? (Is the counselor's role in placement within the agency or district office clearly defined?)
3. Is the counselor aware that there is a perception of less than adequate performance (by the agency, supervisors, or co-workers)?
4. Are there uncontrollable negative factors that might be the cause of poor performance (a particularly difficult or heavy caseload, depressed labor market)?
5. Are there sufficient incentives (rewards) to motivate the counselor to try to improve placement performance? (Is there any reward for quality and quantity of placements made)?

If the answer to any of these questions is "no," then before training is provided, an attempt should be made to correct the problem at this level. If no other reason for performance problems can be isolated and a skill deficiency is found to exist, then an assessment of specific needs can be undertaken.

A well-organized training program will be planned to meet a specific need. To determine training objectives, one must consider the clientele to be served, the new skill or understanding to be realized, and, finally, the program format and instructional method to be employed. To adequately

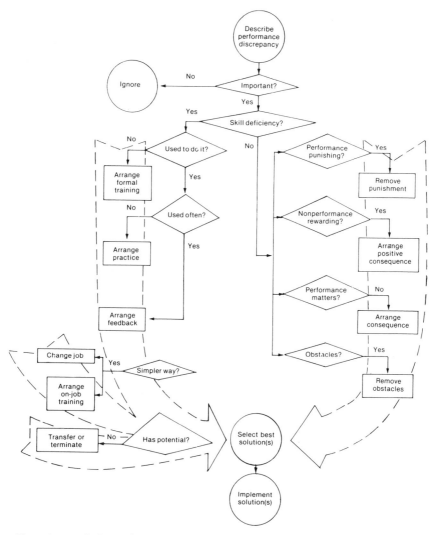

Figure 1.   Analyzing performance problems. (From Mager, R., and Pipe, P. 1970. *Analyzing Performance Problems or "You Really Oughta Wanna,"* p. 100. Fearon Publishers, Belmont, California. By permission.)

and properly plan effective placement training, many people must participate in the program, including administrative and supervisory personnel from the sponsoring program, the trainer, and representatives from the staff to be trained.

The introductory chapter outlines the wide variety of skills that possibly fit under the rubric of job placement activities. All counselors do not need training in all aspects of job placement. Often, either because the role and function of rehabilitation practitioners is unclear or performance evaluations are vague, administrators and supervisors have considerable difficulty in discriminating among the capabilities of their personnel. The result is that training is given, often inappropriately, to a wide section of staff.

Training needs must be established carefully to determine which of the many skills involved in placement must be taught and to whom. Although an assessment of competency in any occupation is a complex and controversial issue, some attempt must be made to establish viable standards to improve performance or close information gaps in any part of the placement process. Fraser and Wright (1977) acknowledged the need for a specific personnel evaluation mechanism and suggested the "Rehabilitation Task Performance Evaluation Scale" as a tool that provides a scale to indicate in which tasks counselors are functioning and at what level of competency. Although still needing increased specificity of performance levels, such an analysis provides agency administration and counselors themselves with a better picture of the array of tasks that constitute the job of the counselor. It also pinpoints the specific areas in which training might be needed in placement.

For example, a "checklist of placement tasks" such as that presented in Table 1 could be used jointly by counselors and supervisors to better define performance expectations and areas in which training may be needed. Does the counselor do job analysis or make employer contacts? If these tasks are not being performed to the degree desired, is this a function of need for skill-building through training, or merely a clearer definition of performance expectations? By better isolating expectations and performance deficits, trainers can develop training programs that meet the information and skill-building needs of individual counselors more precisely. Although such an approach still lacks some precision, it is far superior to current approaches, which force staff to attend training programs that may be inappropriate for their needs. More research is needed to develop instrumentation that would facilitate this assessment process and to explore which tasks contribute most to successful placement.

Developing Training Programs

Rapid development and change in all technical areas makes it necessary for rehabilitation trainers to adopt an interdisciplinary approach to their work. The trainer must be aware of trends in economics, sociology, psychology, and career development in order to provide the information counselors need to place people most effectively. Considering these various disciplines, the trainer can make efficient use of existing information and resources to share with practitioners to aid them in their job of returning rehabilitants to the labor market. Training should also be designed with specific objectives in mind, which aids the trainer to determine whether information alone is sufficient for skill development or whether application of skills is also necessary. For example, do counselors merely need to find out where community resources or major employers are located, or do they need to practice making employer contacts?

The work environment of individuals strongly influences their behavior after a training experience. The trainer, therefore, needs to design training programs with a recognition of the framework within which the individual must operate in the organization. Pre- and post-training efforts must be made to assure that the on-the-job environment is consistent with and, therefore, will reinforce what is attempted in the training session. Otherwise, the effects of change on individuals after they return to work will almost invariably be short lived.

Havelock (1973, pp. 134–136) presents six important conditions which, if established and observed, would ensure the continuance of an innovation. These considerations can be applied to the follow-up needed to ensure that training in placement skills becomes translated to the employee's behavior on the job:

1. *Positive reinforcement*   As previously mentioned, those who receive the training must see that there is a payoff for implementing what they have learned once they are back at work.
2. *Practice and routinization*   Users of an innovation, such as a new office structure to facilitate placement or any new behavior learned through placement training, must be given an opportunity to become familiar with and to try out the innovation repeatedly in the everyday work routine.
3. *Structural integration into the system*   The new behavior or system must become an ongoing part of the work system.
4. *Continuing evaluation*   Some provision should be made for reinspection and reevaluation of the new procedure or innovation over time.
5. *Providing continuing maintenance*   This chiefly involves the need to provide adequate maintenance services when new hardware systems have been introduced (e.g., nothing will dampen enthusiasm more quickly than when job banks are on file in computers that are "down").
6. *Continuing adaptation capability*   There must be ongoing flexibility about altering and modifying procedures as time passes.

If trainers and agency administration work together to ensure that these conditions are taken into consideration as part of an overall training program, the likelihood of training improving placement performance would be expected to be high. A concurrent effort must be made to decide which skills actually promote effective placement and to incorporate new findings into training.

THE ROLE OF AGENCY
ADMINISTRATION IN EFFECTIVE JOB PLACEMENT

Training alone is often not the answer to remediating job performance problems, and training done in isolation will rarely be implemented in the work environment. Rather, training can be a useful complement to an agency's overall effort to enhance placement performance. This section presents discussion on how clarification of the counselor's role and performance expectations in placement, staff and organizational structure, and the agency reward system can influence placement activity.

Relating Training to the Organization

Both organizational development activities and specific staff development efforts focus on making changes that will enhance organizational productivity. The emphasis in organizational management theory has shifted in the last several decades from one that viewed bureaucratic structure as the key to organizational functioning to one that treats the organization as a total system or complex of interdependent subsystems. Successful organizational development is seen as being *system oriented*, concentrating attention not upon units within an organization but on the total system (Aplin and Thompson, 1974).

This approach implies that, since the organizational structure is believed to influence trainees' ability to apply what they have learned, when developing training, trainers of rehabilitation personnel must take into account the characteristics of the organization in which the practitioners actually work. If this systems-oriented view is viable, then not only is it possible to improve organizational functioning through training, but the organizational structure itself can be adapted to better accommodate the new skills and knowledge of counselors.

A systems approach to facilitating placement activity is not a new idea. Burress (1962) states that to be most effective, there must be an organizational structure for conducting placement services in vocational rehabilitation. The organization must also help foster positive attitudes and encourage counselors to skillful performance in placement. According to Beckard (1975), the organization can bring about increased or more effective job placement efforts in the following ways:

1. Change the agency's relationship to the environment (i.e., can the agency more effectively stimulate interest in hiring people with disabilities on the part of employers?)

2. Change the agency's managerial strategy (e.g., top and middle management could take a more active role in job placement)
3. Change the structure of the organization (e.g., add a placement component or placement staff)
4. Change the way the work itself is done (e.g., develop criteria to assess effectiveness)
5. Change the reward system (e.g., the administration ensures that the reward system is consistent with work, rewarding such things as specific placement activities)

All of these are ways for a program to enhance placement efforts. Because they relate more closely to training concerns, clarification of roles, and performance expectations, staff and organizational structure and agency reward systems are discussed in greater detail.

Clarifying the Counselor's Role and Performance Expectations

Poor job performance can be a function of unclear responsibilities. The degree to which counselors are responsible for placement varies not only between VR agencies and rehabilitation facilities but also within agencies of the state/federal system because of differences among supervisors from various district offices. As Chapter 1 points out, the debate over superiority of a placement system involving a generalist counselor as opposed to the use of a placement specialist has yet to be solved. However, failing to make job responsibilities clear and varying performance expectations can lead to unsatisfactory work productivity and lower placement records.

Giblin and Ornati (1977) suggest that not only should employee tasks be clearly outlined, but also that these tasks should be translated into specific outputs or services, which can then be measured. Cook (1977) states that when such output requirements are established cooperatively between workers and management, it is likely that productivity will increase. Organizational management theory thus suggests that improved placement performance might be brought about by clearly specifying the counselor's role in placement. It is also helpful to set up tangible goals for counselor performance within a given period of time. For example, the supervisor and the counselor could, on a monthly or quarterly basis, set goals together on various activities related to the counselor's placement performance (e.g., number of employer contacts made or labor trend information used). Activities to be carried out and final output-placements are expectations that should be clearly defined.

Staff and Organizational Structure and Considerations

Both *whom* the agency hires and *how* they use these personnel can affect overall agency placement performance. Worker productivity is a function not only of a person's skills but also of the relationship among the task itself, the social requirements of the job, and the individual's motivation. Understanding this relationship can help when attempting to improve placement performance. If counselors are not providing placement services in the manner or to the extent to which administration believes possible, then staff motivation and the interaction of task and social variables may need to be assessed.

Some counselors may have negative attitudes toward or a fear of engaging in placement activities and, therefore, it may be futile for an agency to attempt to force them to do so (Dunn, 1974). Rather, sound staff development approaches should attempt to focus on and make maximum use of the skills and interests of these existing staff, perhaps using training reinforcement, support staff, reorganization of program structure, promotional opportunities, or other possible performance motivators to improve attitudes toward the placement function. Staff hiring criteria might also be adopted to aid administration to better identify new employees who would be good placement counselors.

Problems may arise if placement training is provided for only one level of staff (Molinaro, 1977). All levels of staff must be aware of the goals of placement training and, if not personally involved in planning or receiving training themselves, their support of the training should be assured. Ideally, supervisory staff should be able to assume placement responsibilities themselves, verifying the importance of placement in the rehabilitation process. The role of the VR supervisor is critical to the success of implementation of newly learned skills on the job. There is no doubt that leadership and supervision in the work environment have an important impact on the motivation, commitment, adaptability, and satisfaction of employees (Huse and Beer, 1971). Supervisory staff should be involved, whenever possible, in the development, presentation, and follow-up of inservice placement training.

The comparatively small amount of the time spent in placement activity discovered by Muthard and Salomone (1969) appears to remain unchanged for the VR caseload-carrying counselor today. Zadny and James (1977) reported that counselors spend only about 3 hours per week (7% of their time) on placement, based on survey data gathered from over 200 caseload-carrying counselors. Lillehaugen (1964) suggested that low placement activity could be attributed to the heavy caseloads and administrative duties of counselors, and that special placement counselors might be the answer to the problem of time devoted to placement. These special counselors would be expected to spend one-half of their time contacting employers and the other half coordinating job placement for clients. This concept was later more fully developed by Hutchinson and Cogan (1974), who described the role and function of a "rehabilitation manpower specialist" in strengthening an agency's placement efforts. Usdane (1976) presented the array of skills and information that such a placement person should have in order to carry out programs concerning job development, job solicitation, economic job forecasting, labor market information, job engineering, and job information.

Placement specialists have not been universally employed by VR agencies for a variety of reasons. It is not the purpose of this chapter to build a case for their use, but rather to urge strongly that agencies assess whether size of caseloads and complexity of the labor market, particularly in many large urban areas, does not require a change in staff organization so that certain counselors could spend more time in placement. Low placement activity may not be a matter of lack of placement skills, but rather may be attributed to an insufficient amount of time spent on using acquired skills.

In addition to hiring and a need for staff supervisory support, placement performance in a program can also be enhanced by efficient office organization. A systematic and well-organized approach to developing job leads and matching them to people ready to work seems to be particularly needed in large metropolitan areas. Molinaro (1977) described the development and implementation of a selective job placement system in the Michigan VR agency, where a number of specialized units in the system (i.e., account system, job bank, skill bank, and employer services) were created to facilitate both job development and job placement. Not all of these specialized units are needed to have a successful placement program. It is important, however, for an agency to assess the placement training needs of its staff while exploring alterations or additions to office structure that might improve the overall placement effort.

Rewarding Placement Performance

An organization that wants its worker to perform in a certain manner must create ways of organizing a reward system that will encourage better staff performance. There are several ways in which rewards could be built into the VR system to encourage more and better placements.

Placement performance has historically been measured by counting up numbers of people placed in jobs in terms of increases in earnings. However, Dunn (1974) has suggested that program effectiveness should be examined in greater detail. Although sheer number might suggest that vocational rehabilitation has been effective in finding jobs for people with disabilities, Dunn pointed out that state agency rehabilitants tend to be placed in unskilled industrial and service occupations more frequently than the rest of the labor force as a whole. Those with disabilities are underrepresented in professional, skilled, and semi-skilled occupations.

Giblin and Ornati (1977) suggest that it is more likely that an organization will make maximum use of its work force when the rewards (i.e., wages and career opportunities) correspond to both the quality and the quantity of the worker's output. Historically, in the state agencies, only a 26 closure has been thought of as a "successful rehabilitation"; no emphasis has been placed on the *quality* of employment itself (e.g., promotional opportunities). This view of success is also found in rehabilitation facilities. As the introductory chapter suggests, however, the quality of rehabilitation services could be monitored by assessing both financial and nonmonetary rewards that an individual receives because of VR services. Backer (1977) affirms that administrators in state VR agencies and private settings can do much to implement revised and improved systems of outcome measurement. These systems can serve usefully not only for individual counselor self-improvement and performance appraisal but can also provide useful information for overall program improvement. More simply, the agency could recognize distinctions in the quality of placements based on whether they were made in the primary or secondary labor markets. This judgment, of course, would have to depend on the levels of productivity a person actually brings to the labor market. If counselors were motivated by checks on the quality of their placements, it is highly likely that appropriateness of placements would improve.

Concrete rewards related to performance and an overall atmosphere of support and reinforcement are necessary if an agency wants to encourage improved placement performance on the part of its staff. Most workers will respond with energy and effort when they see that placement activity is considered valuable by their organization, supervisors, and co-workers.

CONCLUSION

Program administrators, rehabilitation trainers, and educators need to develop and be aware of the spectrum of skills that improve the placement performance of a vocational rehabilitation counselor. Rehabilitation counselor education programs can better provide future counselors with the general information and skills they need to begin placement activity once on the job. Agency administration and training staff must decide which placement skills counselors need to have and determine which personnel members need training in specific skill areas.

Traditional approaches to training, staff development planning, and implementation must be abandoned for a new approach, which considers both the specific needs of the learner and those of the organization. The burden of responsibility for good training rests with program administration and rehabilitation trainers. The administrative plan must consist of an approach that will encourage openness to change and development on the part of both the individual staff person and that of the agency as a whole. By developing and implementing a total agency placement effort, an administration can create conditions under which individuals are able to use their skills to effectively place individuals with disabilities into the labor market.

REFERENCES

Aplin, J. C., and Thompson, D. E. 1974. Successful organizational change. Bus. Horizons 12(4):61–66.

Backer, T. E. 1977. New Directions in Rehabilitation Outcome Measurement. Institute for Research Utilization, Washington, D.C.

Beckard, R. 1975. Strategies for large system change. Sloan Manage. Rev. 16(2):43–55.

Burress, J. R. 1962. Placement services lag in vocational rehabilitation. J. Rehab. 28(4):28.

Cook, D. C. 1977. Would you trust your workers with a decision? Indust. Week 194(3):51–54.

Dunn, D. J. 1974. Placement Services in the Vocational Rehabilitation Program. University of Wisconsin—Stout Vocational Rehabilitation Institute Research and Training Center, Menomonie, Wisconsin.

Fraser, R. T., and Wright, G. N. 1977. Improving rehabilitation personnel management. J. Rehab. 43(3):22–24.

Giblin, E. J., and Ornati, O. A. 1977. Optimizing the utilization of human resources. J. Rehab. Admin. 1(2):4–13.

Havelock, R. G. 1973. The Change Agent's Guide to Innovation in Education. Educational Technology Publications, Englewood Cliffs, New Jersey.

Huse, E. F., and Beer, M. 1971. Eclectic approach to organizational development. Harvard Bus. Rev. Sept.–Oct.: 103–112.

Hutchinson, J., and Cogan, E. 1974. Rehabilitation manpower specialist: A job description of placement personnel. J. Rehab. 40(2):31–33.

Jaques, M. E. 1959. Critical counseling behavior in rehabilitation settings. State University of Iowa, College of Education, Iowa City.

Lillehaugen, S. T. 1964. District placement counselors can boost jobs for handicapped. Rehab. Rec. 5(2):29–31.

Mager, R. F., and Pipe, P. 1970. Analyzing Performance Problems or "You Really Oughta Wanna." Fearon Publishers, Belmont, California.

Molinaro, D. 1977. A placement system develops and settles: The Michigan model. Rehab. Counsel. Bull. 21(2):121–129.

Muthard, J. E., and Salomone, P. R. 1969. The roles and functions of rehabilitation counselors. Rehab. Counsel. Bull. 13(1).

Scorzelli, J. F. 1975. Reactions to program content of a rehabilitation counseling program. J. Appl. Rehab. Counsel. 6(3):172–177.

Usdane, W. M. 1976. The placement process in the rehabilitation of the severely disabled. Rehab. Lit. 37(6):162–167.

Usdane, W. M. 1977. Comments: Subsidized extended employment plus intensive placement activity. Rehab. Lit. 38(4):188–119.

Wright, G. N., and Fraser, R. T. 1976. Improving Manpower Utilization: The Rehabilitation Task Performance Evaluation Scale. Wisconsin Studies in Vocational Rehabilitation. University of Wisconsin Rehabilitation Research Institute, Madison.

Zadny, J. J., and James, L. F. 1977. Job Placement of the Vocationally Handicapped. Part V—Counselor Technique and Placement Performance: Placement Assistance, Contacting Employers, Monitoring and Follow-up and Caseload Management. Portland State University Studies in Placement and Job Development for the Handicapped, Monograph 2. Portland State University School of Social Work, Portland, Oregon.

Index